Advances in Biomedical Corrosion:

Trends, Challenges, and Solutions

Edited by Jean L. Broge

AMPP™

AMPP

Association for Materials Protection and Performance

Cover image courtesy of Getty Images.

ISBN Print: 978-1-57590-488-7

ISBN PDF: 978-1-57590-489-4

Neither AMPP, its officers, directors, nor members thereof accept any responsibility for the use of the methods and materials discussed herein. No authorization is implied concerning the use of patented or copyrighted material. The information is advisory only and the use of the materials and methods is solely at the risk of the user.

AMPP

Association for Materials Protection and Performance
15835 Park Ten Place
Houston, TX 77084

Table of Contents

From the Editor

Advances in Biomedical Corrosion: Trends, Challenges, and Solutions is a collection of 10+ years of research in the biomedical field specific to corrosion, be it in materials development or manufacturing processes.

While biomedical materials can be made from a wide range of materials including metals, alloys, ceramics, and polymers, each with its own corrosion susceptibility and behavior, this compilation focuses on metals and alloys.

For those who want a refresher or want to learn more, or anything, about biomedical corrosion, it is also known as biomedical materials corrosion or biocorrosion. The term refers to the process of deterioration or degradation of materials used in biomedical applications due to interactions within biological environments. The corrosion of medical devices and implants is, of course, a major concern as the corrosion of such materials can lead to various adverse effects, including implant failure, tissue damage, and systemic health issues.

The main factors influencing corrosion in biomedical applications are the specific biological environment, material composition, design, and the presence of mechanical forces or stresses. Here are some key points about biomedical corrosion:

Types of Corrosion: Biomedical materials can experience distinct types of corrosion, including uniform corrosion, localized corrosion (such as pitting and crevice corrosion), galvanic corrosion, and stress corrosion cracking.

Biological Environment: In the human body, biomedical materials are exposed to a complex environment containing various chemical species, electrolytes, enzymes, proteins, and cells. The pH, temperature, and presence of corrosive substances can vary depending on the location of the implant or medical device.

Metallic Implants: Metals and alloys used in orthopedic implants (*e.g.*, stainless steel, titanium alloys, cobalt-chromium alloys) are susceptible to corrosion due to the aggressive nature of physiological fluids, leading to ion release and implant deterioration.

Corrosion of Dental Materials: Dental implants and restorative materials are also susceptible to corrosion in the oral environment, which contains saliva, acids, and several types of bacteria.

Protective Measures: To mitigate biomedical corrosion, researchers and manufacturers employ various protective measures, such as using corrosion-resistant materials, surface coatings (*e.g.*, titanium oxide coatings on titanium implants), and biocompatible materials that promote tissue integration.

Biodegradable Materials: In some cases, biomedical materials are intentionally designed to be biodegradable, gradually degrading in the body as new tissue forms, reducing the need for removal surgeries.

Testing and Standards: Biomedical materials undergo extensive testing to assess their corrosion resistance and biocompatibility before approval for clinical use. Several international standards and guidelines exist to ensure the safety and performance of these materials.

Long-term Effects: Long-term corrosion of biomedical materials can result in the release of metal ions into the body, potentially causing local inflammation, allergic reactions, or systemic health issues.

Suffice to say, all the above are covered within these pages.

It should be understood as well that regular monitoring of implanted materials is essential to detect any signs of corrosion-related issues and ensure patient safety.

Paper Number:
C2012-01510

Crevice Corrosion of Biomedical Alloys: A Novel Method of Assessing the Effects of Bone Cement and Its Chemistry

M. Bryant
Institute of Engineering Thermofluids

X. Hu
Institute of Engineering Thermofluids

R. Farrar
DePuy International Ltd, Leeds

K. Brummitt
DePuy International Ltd, Leeds

R. Freeman
DePuy International Ltd, Leeds

A. Neville
Institute of Engineering Thermofluids

Abstract

Studies to date have identified that the introduction of antibiotics into PMMA bone cement can affect the crevice corrosion initiation and propagation mechanisms of commonly used biomaterials. In this study, five commercially available Poly(methyl methacrylate) PMMA bone cements were tested to investigate the effects of antibiotics on the severity of crevice corrosion. Bone cements with varying chemistry were also tested. A test method was developed in part reference to ASTM F746-04. Cylindrical specimens were fitted with a bone cement tapered collar, creating consistent crevice conditions. Crevice corrosion was then studied using potentiodynamic polarization technique in deaerated phosphate buffered saline solution (pH7.4) at 37°C. Surface analyses using a light microscope and scanning electron microscopy (SEM) were also conducted to investigate the surface morphology after accelerated electrochemical testing. Initial testing of commercially-available bone cements indicated that different PMMA bone cements can affect the initiation and propagation mechanism of crevice corrosion. Further studies have identified that the addition of radiopaque agent and antibiotics affect the initiation mechanisms in 316L stainless steel, whilst significantly increasing the extent of propagation in CoCrMo alloys.

Keywords: crevice corrosion, biomaterials, bone cement, CoCrMo and 316L stainless steel, ion release

INTRODUCTION

In vivo, the human body is a harsh chloride-containing biological environment, lending itself to the accelerated dissolution of alloys and the release of potentially toxic metal ions. Corrosion of biomedical implants is a complex multi-factorial process depending on implant design, metallurgy, mechanical interactions and solution chemistry.[1] During Total Hip Arthroplasty (THA), the medullary canal is reamed to size using a series or reamers and rasps and a PMMA cement restrictor placed at the bottom of the canal and the cement is introduced and pressurized in a retrograde fashion. The femoral stem is then introduced into the cement, until the desired position is met and the remaining cement cleaned away to leave the bone cement mantle. This introduction of the stem into the bone cement has been shown to result in interactions both undesirable from a mechanical loading and electrochemical point of view.

The Ultima TPS™ hip replacement system (DePuy International, Leeds) was developed to be one of the first 2nd generation cemented metal-on-metal total hip replacements, introduced in 1997 as a modular femoral stem, typically used in patients with structural damage. Modularity of this type allowed a surgeon the opportunity to select compo-

Figure 1

Ultima TPS™ metal-on-metal hip replacement retrieval showing evidence of corrosion at the proximal stem-cement interface and the distal stem surface (arrows).

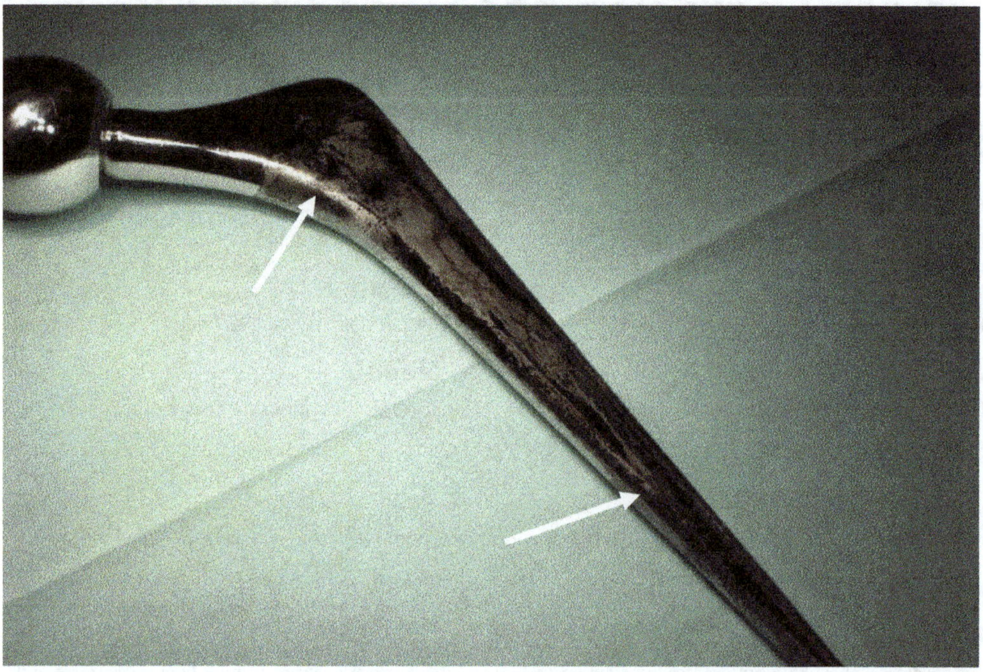

nents most suited to patients' anatomical and functional needs. The highly polished low carbon CoCrMo tapered stem was designed to accommodate cement creep and self-locking in the antero-posterior and medio-lateral planes.

In 2008, 90 out of a total series of 652 The Ultima TPS™ metal-on-metal hip replacements had to undergo early revision at the Norfolk and Norwich University Hospital.[2] 17 hips required revision for periprosthetic fracture, with early dislocation in 3 and late dislocations in 16. Infection was found in 10 hips. 44 required revision for extensive, symptomatic, peri-articular soft tissue necrosis of which 35 had normal plain radiographs. Dramatic corrosion of generally solidly fixed femoral stems was frequently observed on the retrieved cemented part of the femoral component (Figure 1).[2] It was thought that the necrosis of the surrounding tissue was associated with the release of potentially toxic metal ions such as cobalt and chromium from the stem surface.[2]

A similar case has also been reported by *Bolland et al* describing localized corrosion of a similar collarless polished tapered cobalt chromium stem (CPT; Zimmer, Warsaw, Indiana), implanted with antibiotic bone cement (Heraeus Medical GMbH, Hanau, Germany).[3] *Bolland* described that the stem had obvious pitting and evidence of corrosion along the surface which was more marked at the region of the proximal cement/stem interface and the tip of the stem (Figure 2), similar to the characteristics presented by *Donell et al.*[2] At retrieval a large volume of necrotic tissue in the cement-bone interface had occurred. Resorption and cortical thinning had also occurred resulting in pathological fracture. High levels of Co in whole blood samples were observed in the cohort awaiting revision, however no significant levels of Cr and Mo were noted.

Figure 2

Explanted collarless polished tapered cobalt chromium stem showing evidence of corrosion at the proximal stem-cement interface and the distal stem surface (arrows). [3]

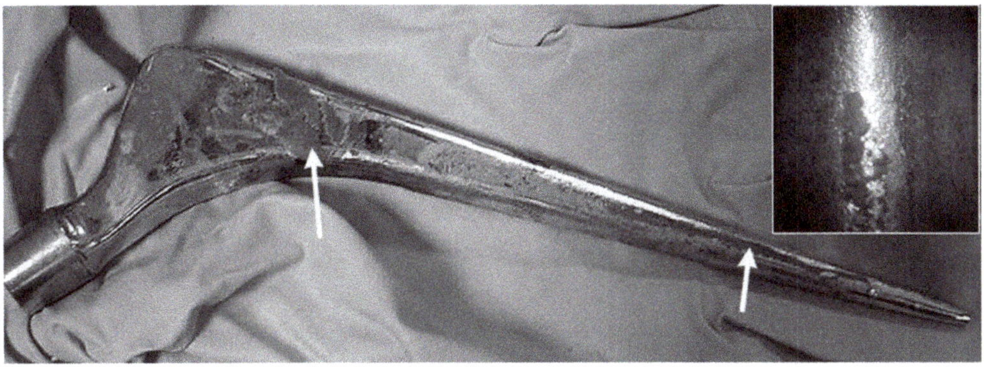

Although crevice corrosion of cemented THR has been identified in retrieval studies by authors as a failure mechanism, studies into the effects of bone cement and cementing technique on crevice corrosion have not yet been investigated.[2-5]

The integration of antibiotics in PMMA bone cements for the treatment and prevention of infection in orthopedics has become common clinical practice since the 1970's, with gentamicin sulphate been extensively used as the primary antibiotic.[6, 7] However, studies to date have questioned the efficacy of the use of antibiotic impregnated cements as the release mechanisms are poorly understood and difficult to control whilst maintaining the integrity of the implant.[7] Similarly, questions around how antibiotics and radiopaque agents affect the localized corrosion regimes of cemented implants need to be answered. Although crevice corrosion has been extensively studied to address a wide range of industrial issues, there has been no application of the mechanisms and models applied to clinical aspects. This paper presents how the additions of antibiotic and radiopaque agents affect the initiation and propagation mechanisms of localized crevice corrosion of commonly used biomaterials.

TEST METHOD & MATERIALS

In this study a crevice geometry was adapted from ASTM 746-04 to study the crevice corrosion of biomaterials used in THR. A cylindrical specimen, with a diameter of 6 ± 0.1 mm, length of 20 ± 0.1 mm and an average surface roughness of $R_a = 0.2$ μm were fitted with a bone cement tapered collar to create a crevice with an opening of approx 0.4 ± 0.1 mm and crevice volume of 7.70 mm^3 (Figure 3). A three electrode electrochemical cell was utilized consisting of the crevice assembly as the working electrode and a Thermo Scientific Sureflow Redox combination electrode, consisting of a Ag/AgCl reference electrode and Pt counter electrode, in order to simulate accelerated electrochemical corrosion. A schematic representation of the experimental setup can be seen in Figure 4. The assembly was then immersed in deaerated phosphate buffered saline solution at 37±1°C until the rest potential had stabilized to a rate of change less than 3 mV/min. Crevice corrosion was then simulated by conducting potentiodynamic polarization scans. The potentiodynamic scan was started 300mV below the free corrosion potential (E_{corr}), with the potential being shifted in the noble or positive direction at a scan rate of 0.167 mV/Sec. The scan was then reversed when the current density reaches approximately 500 μA/cm^2. The reverse scan was stopped when the

Figure 3

Tapered washer artificial crevice design.

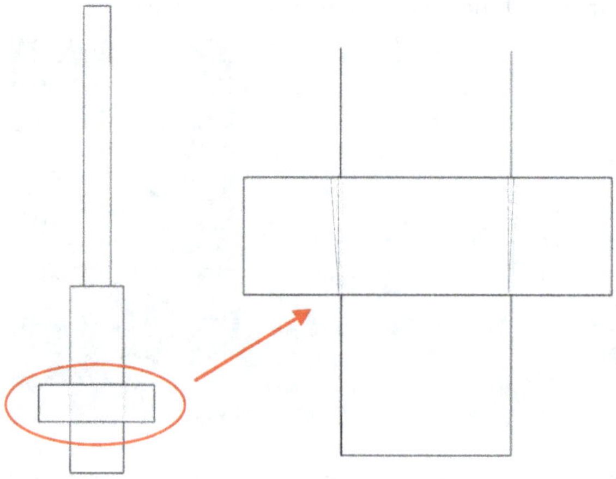

Figure 4

3-D modelling of the crevice corrosion cell.

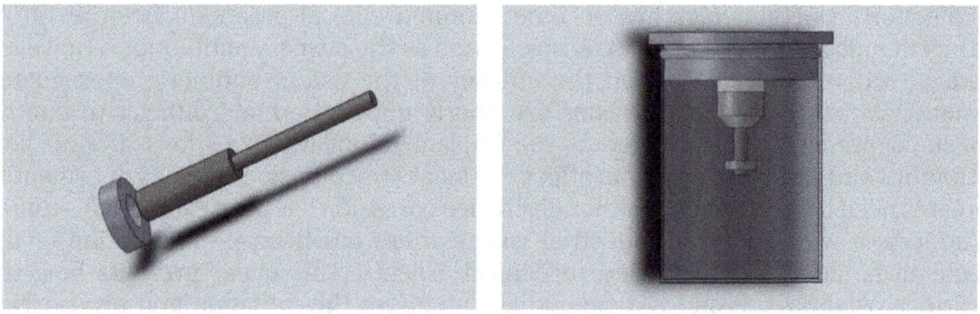

current had become less than that of forward scan. The free corrosion potential (E_{corr}), breakdown potential (E_b) and repassivation potential (E_r) were used to characterize a materials resistance to electrochemical corrosion of commonly used biomaterials. Definition of these parameters can be found in Figure 5. For the 316 L stainless steel samples breakdown potential was taken at $10\mu A/cm^2$; a current density described by Oldfield and Sutton considered enough to cause permanent breakdown of the passive film.[8] For CoCrMo samples, breakdown was taken by extrapolating the active and passive regions and taking the point of intersect. Optical microscope analysis and scanning electron microscopy (SEM) were utilized as a method of observing the surface morphology after accelerated electrochemical tests.

During this study two commonly used biomaterials were investigated. Low carbon CoCrMo (BS ISO 5832-12) and 316L stainless steel (BS ISO 5832-1) were used in *in-vitro* corrosion tests. Initially, five commercially available PMMA bone cements (Table 1) were tested according to the protocol outlined below. In addition, cement variation tests to assess the effect of antibiotic concentration and radiopaque agents with respect to localized crevice corrosion were conducted. A PMMA base powder was taken and varying levels of gentamacin sulphate, barium sulphate and zirconium dioxide added (Table 2). Each powder component was passed through a 60 mesh sieve, placed in

Figure 5

Schematic of a Polarization plot with studied parameters.

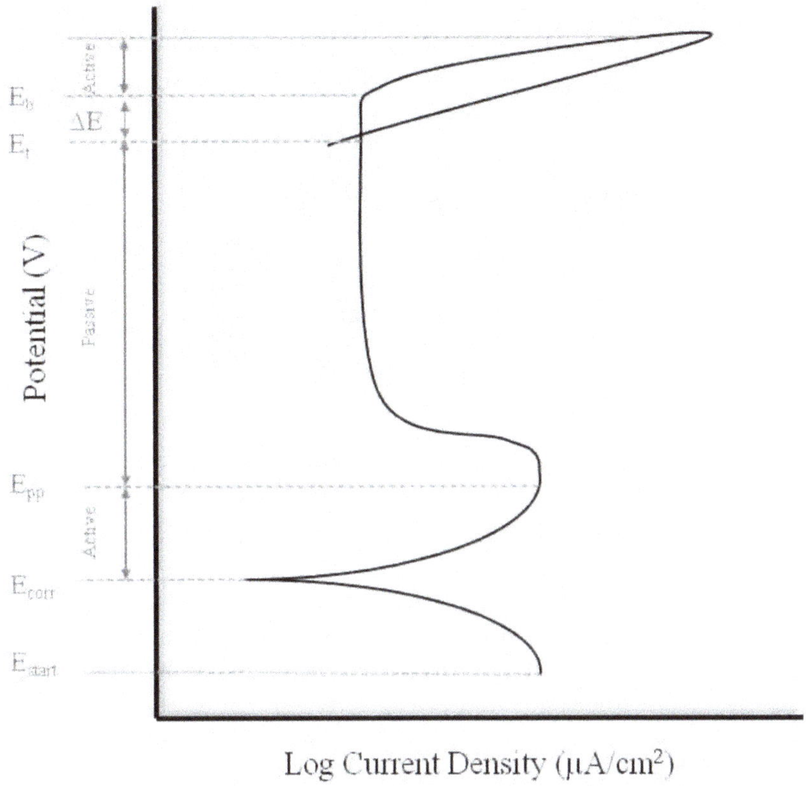

a polythene liner and then blended for ten minutes. The powder blend and liquid monomer components were mixed at an approximate ratio of 2:1 to form PMMA cement rods. Each rod was then machined to create the bone cement tapered collars.

This particular test is a modification of the established ASTM F746 – 04 standard and was used as a screening to rank cement and implant alloy combination in order of their resistance to localized corrosion.[9] This test method only applies to passive

Table 1

Commercially available tested cements in this study.

Cement ID	Bone Cement
NA_1	Non antibiotic with barium sulphate
NA_2	Non antibiotic with zirconium dioxide
AB_1	Gentamicin sulphate (4.22% w/w) with zirconium dioxide
AB_2	Gentamicin sulphate (1.96% w/w) with zirconium dioxide
AB_3	Erythromycin (as glucoheptonate) & colistin sulphomethate sodium (1.21% w/w Erythromycin & 3.00 million I.U Colistin) with barium sulphate

Figure 6

E_{corr} when stabilized to a rate of change ≤ 3mV/sec for 316L stainless steel with commercially-available bone cements.

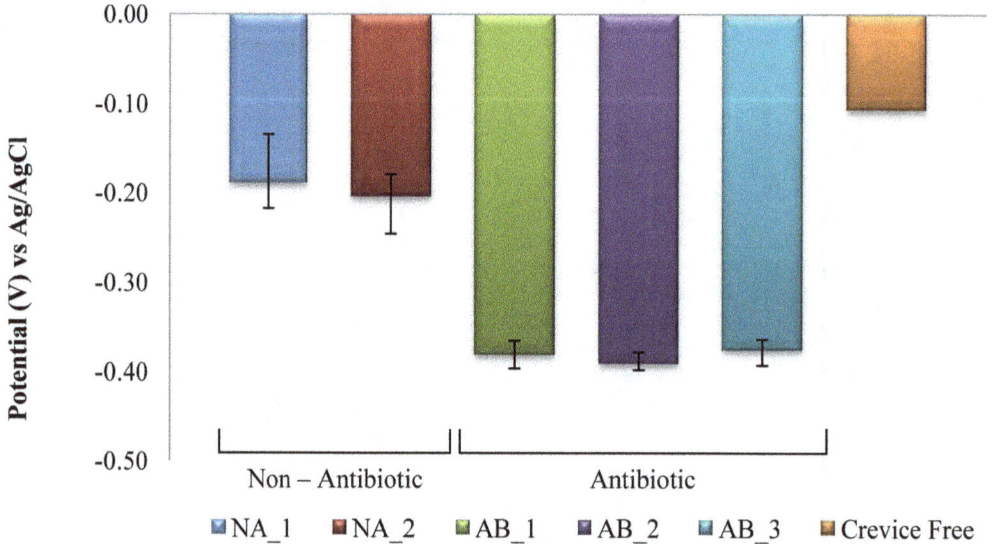

metals and alloys as non-passive materials are considered inappropriate as implantable materials. It is important to note that these particular tests did not take into account any processes that take place at the cement interface during the cementing process.

RESULTS

Commercially-Available Cements

Figure 6 demonstrates the free corrosion potential (E_{corr}) for 316L stainless steel samples when the sample E_{corr} had stabilized to a rate of change less than 3 mV/min. It can be seen that samples combined with cements containing antibiotic had a much more negative E_{corr} compared to samples combined with non-antibiotic cements. The more negative potential is considered to be associated with a materials tendency

Table 2

Concentrations of self-prepared cements.

Base Powder	Additions Powder
40g PMMA	N/A
40g PMMA	1.68g Gentamicin sulphate
40g PMMA	3.36g Gentamicin sulphate
40g PMMA	4g Barium sulphate
40g PMMA	10g Barium sulphate
40g PMMA	6g Zirconium dioxide
40g PMMA	12g Zirconium dioxide

Figure 7

E_b of 316L with commercially-available bone cements at a current density of 10μA/cm^2.

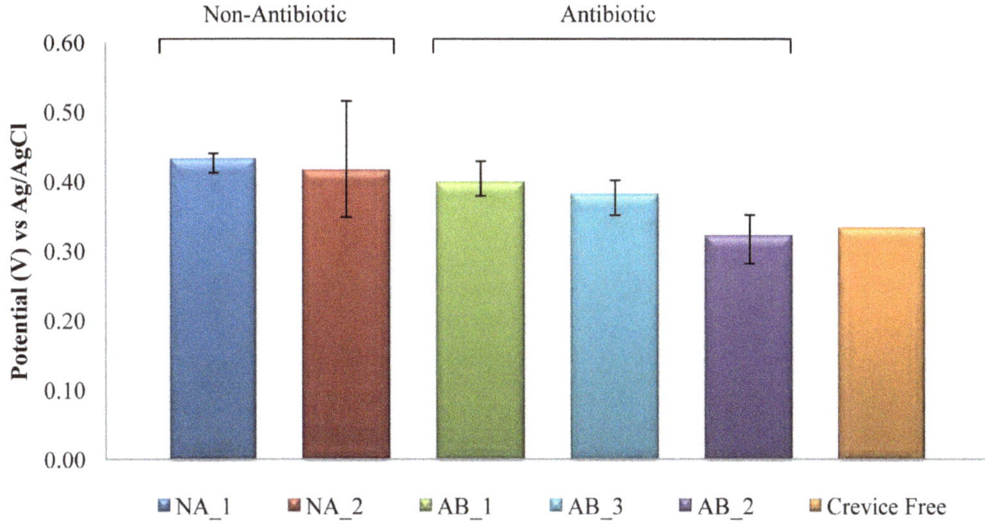

corrode. These results would suggest that when a stainless steel specimen is combined with NA_1 and NA_2 bone cement, the tendency for that specimen to corrode is less, compared to samples combined with antibiotic cement.

The results from the initial open circuit potential results were further strengthened by the breakdown potential (E_b) measurements. Breakdown potential was taken to be the potential at the current density of 10μA/cm^2, which is considered to be the point at which complete breakdown of the passive film occurs for 316L stainless steel.[10] Figure 7 demonstrates the measurements obtained from the Potentiodynamic curves. It can be seen that the cements containing antibiotics demonstrated a lower breakdown potential, indicating that the antibiotic in the bone cement increases the susceptibility to localized corrosion for 316L. 316L stainless steel combined with NA_1 bone cement had the highest resistance to localized corrosion, compared to AB_3, which demonstrated the lowest resistance to localized crevice corrosion.

Metastable current peaks were also observed during the potentiodynamic polarization tests. This indicates that the spontaneous formation and repassivation of active localized corrosion was occurring before complete breakdown of the passive film. It could be seen that that the samples combined with non-antibiotic bone cement exhibited an increased amount of metastable events before complete film dissolution.

A similar trend was also observed for the low carbon CoCrMo samples. Figure 8 demonstrates the initial open circuit potential measurements for CoCrMo samples when the rate of change in E_{corr} was ≤3mV/sec. It can be seen that the initial E_{corr} was more negative for the cements containing antibiotic with the exception of the AB_1 cement. Although E_{corr} measurements are of a semi-quantitative nature, this would suggest that the AB_2 and AB_3 cements create an initial environment preferential to localized crevice corrosion. Samples without the tapered washer were also analyzed as a control to ensure crevice corrosion was occurring. It was seen that the E_{corr} for

Figure 8

E_{corr} when stabilized to a rate of change ≤ 3mV/sec for CoCrMo with commercially-available bone cements.

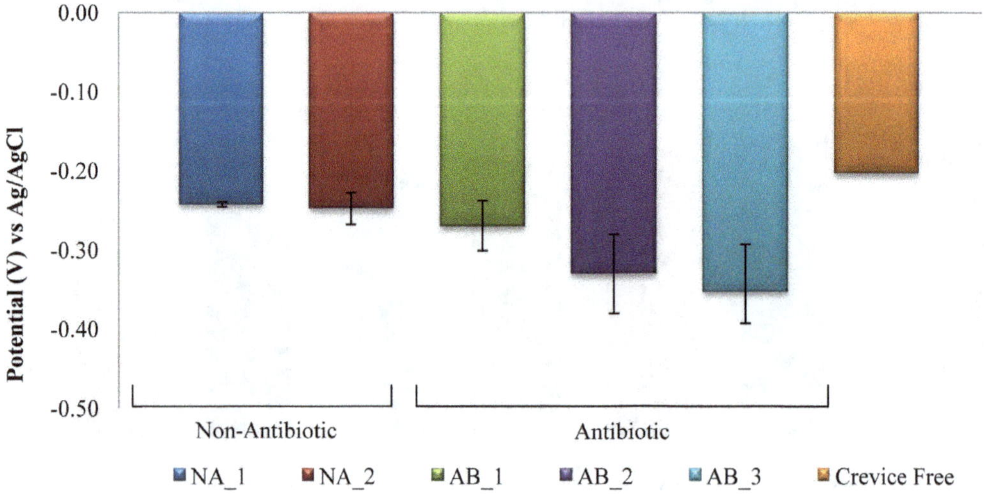

Figure 9

E_b of low carbon CoCrMo with commercially-available bone cements.

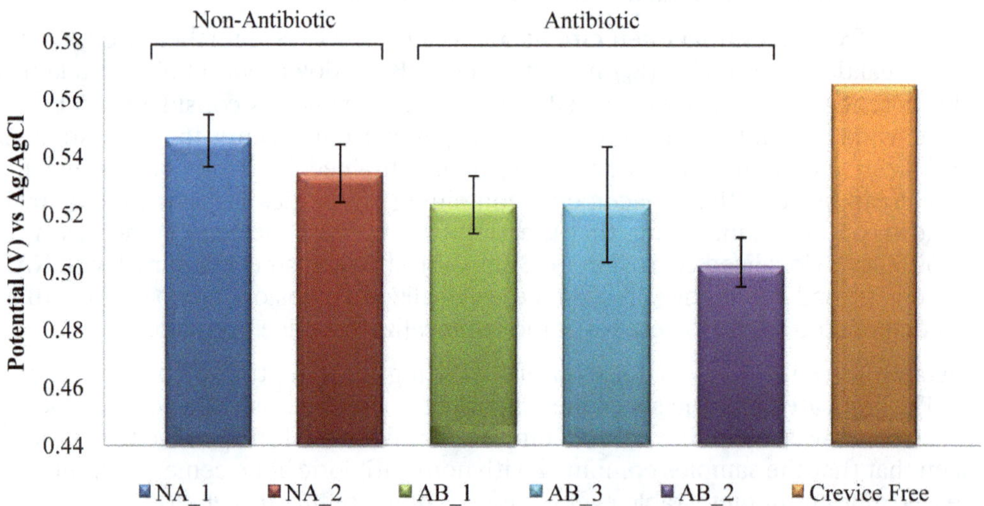

the 'crevice free' samples was more positive than the samples fitted with the tapered washer, indicating that samples fitted with the washers had an increased tendency to localized corrosion.

The results obtained from the polarization curves again confirmed the E_{corr} measurements. A similar trend to the stainless steel samples was noted for the CoCrMo samples. A decrease in breakdown potential was seen for samples combined with antibiotic cement, with samples combined with AB_2 cement displaying the worst susceptibility to localized crevice corrosion. Figure 9 demonstrates the breakdown potentials

Figure 10

E_r of low carbon CoCrMo with commercially-available bone cements.

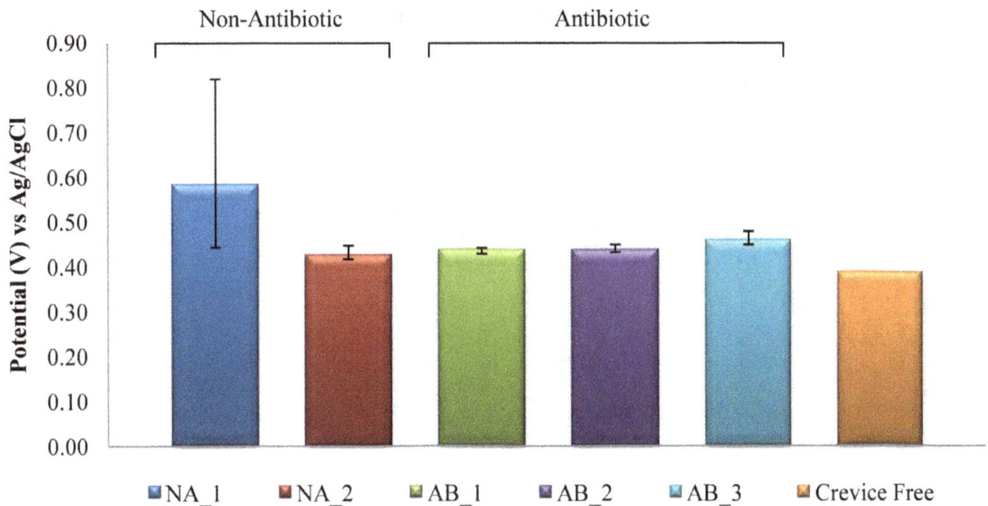

for CoCrMo specimens. Samples not fitted with a tapered collar demonstrated an increased breakdown potential, demonstrating that CoCrMo can be susceptible to localized crevice corrosion.

Figure 10 demonstrates the repassivation potential values obtained for the CoCrMo specimens. The re-passivation potential represents the potential at which the passive film completely reforms during the reverse scan, deeming the surface of the material once again passive. It can be seen that samples combined with NA_1 bone cement demonstrated an increased re-passivation potential, compared to the remaining samples. Figure 10 indicates that CoCrMo specimens combined with NA_2, AB_1, AB_2 and AB_3 had a similar repassivation potential, with the 'un-creviced' specimen demonstrating the lowest repassivation potential. This suggests that the extent of corrosion was increased on samples not fitted with the tapered bone cement collar; however, these results alone are ambiguous with respect to the propagation of localized crevice corrosion.

Surface analysis of the samples was also carried out to quantify the type of corrosion on the surface of the materials. Initiation and propagation of localized corrosion was seen on the 316L samples, with a macroscopically difference being seen between the samples combined with the antibiotic cement. Figures 11 and 12 demonstrate the optical images taken on 316L after polarization.

Scanning Electron Microscopy (SEM) images indicated a thick layer of corrosion was present on the surface of samples combined with NA_1, NA_2 and AB_1 cements (Figure 13). Area 'A', on Figure 14 demonstrates the surface outside of the crevice, area 'B' demonstrates the surface within the crevice. It is clear to see that a substantial amount of electrochemical damage has occurred as a result of localized crevice corrosion. Intergranular corrosion was also visible on all of the 316L specimens (Figure 15) apart from specimens combined with the NA_2 cement. In all cases SEM analysis indicated that localized crevice corrosion had occurred, with clear and visible areas of localized crevice corrosion being observed on each 316L stainless steel sample.

Figure 11

316L Stainless steel with NA_1 cement.

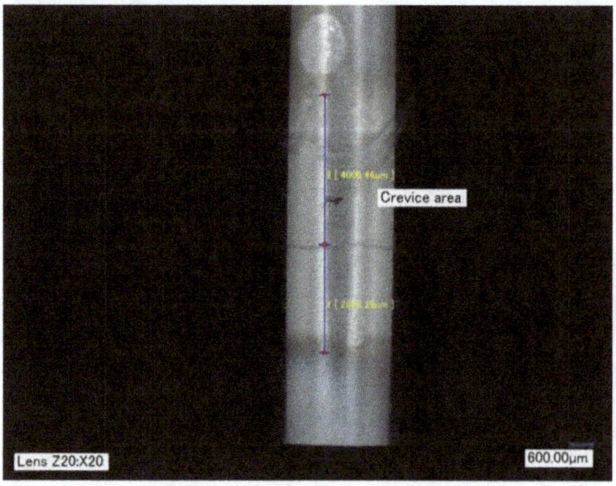

Figure 12

316L Stainless steel with AB_3 cement.

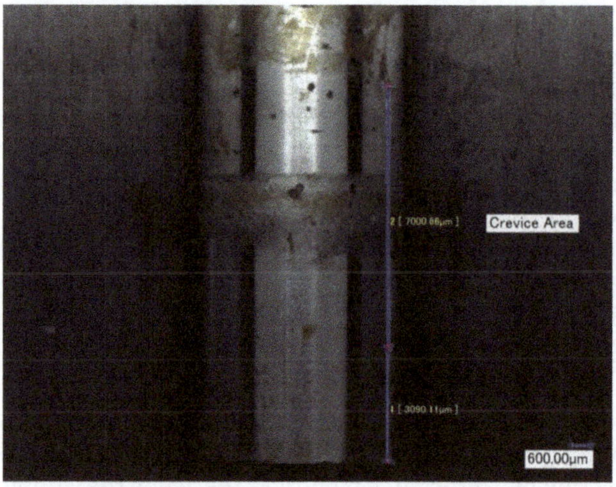

SEM analysis was also conducted on the CoCrMo samples. However, the extent of localized corrosion was not as great due to the higher integrity of the alloy. The enhanced localized corrosion resistance results from a more tenacious oxide film compared to 316L, primarily due to the higher Cr content. Small areas of localized pitting were also noted. SEM images complement the results that were obtained in the electrochemical measurements.

Cement Variation Tests

Cement variation tests were also conducted using the same test method to investigate the effects of different additives in PMMA base bone cement. Parameters tested are outlined in Table 2. Figure 18 demonstrates the breakdown potentials that were obtained for the 316L alloy. Results indicate that the addition of antibiotic and radiopaque

Figure 13

Corrosion product within the 316L and AB_1 bone cement crevice.

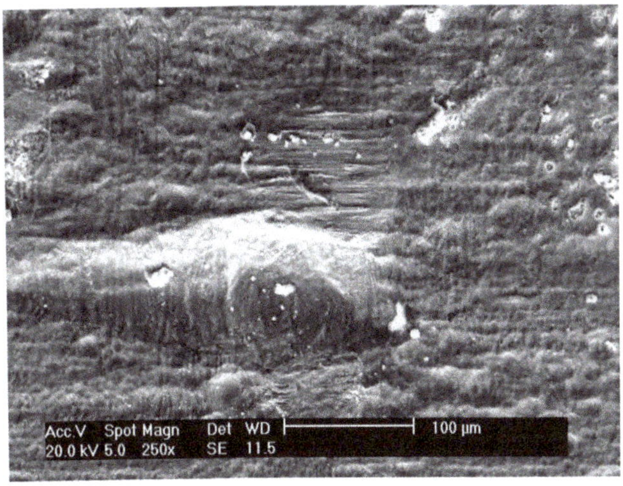

Figure 14

Crevice corrosion profile of the NA_1 samples.

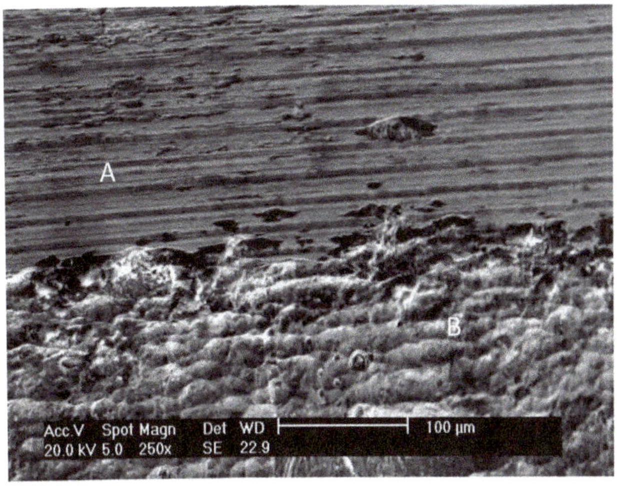

agent can affect the initiation mechanisms of 316L Stainless steel thus reducing the passivity of the alloy. A decrease from 0.324V to 0.219V was observed when 10g barium sulphate was added to the bone cement. It is worth noting that this is around double of that found in commercially available bone cements. However, a decrease from 0.324V to 0.296V was observed when 4g of barium sulphate was added to the base cement.

Due to the increased passive nature of the CoCrMo, the addition of antibiotics and radiopaque agent had no significant effect on the passivity of the material. However, it was observed that propagation mechanisms of localized corrosion were affected with the addition of antibiotics and radiopaques agents. Propagation of localized corrosion was characterized by, and described as ΔE ($\Delta E = E_b - E_r$). Figure 19 demonstrates the

Figure 15

Intergranular corrosion of 316L with AB_1 cement.

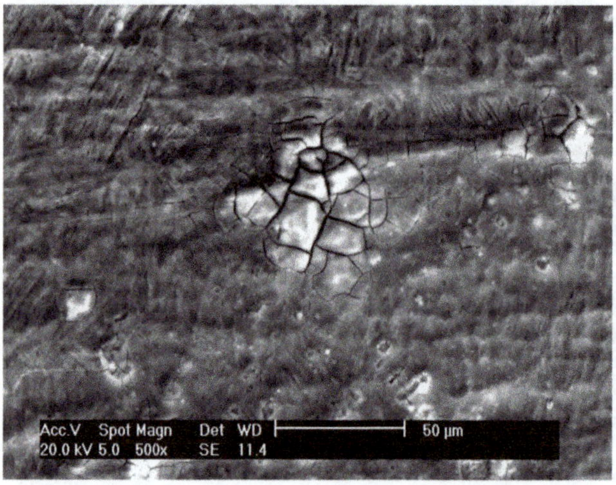

Figure 16

SEM image of corrosion product within the CoCrMo and AB_1 bone cement crevice.

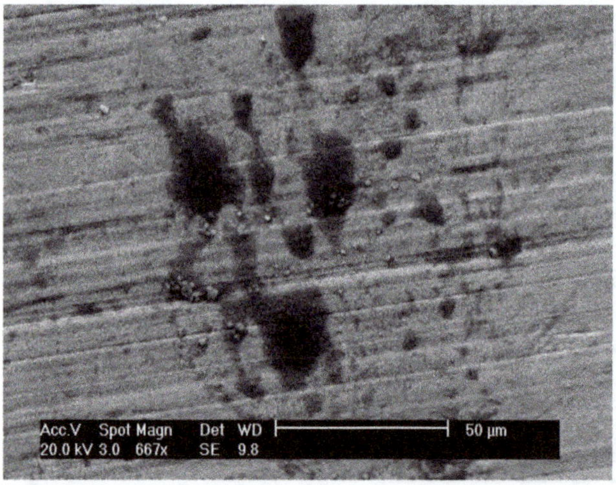

ΔE values that were obtained from the CoCrMo samples. When compared with the base PMMA cement the addition of radiopaque agent and antibiotics was seen to influence the propagation mechanisms of localized corrosion.

DISCUSSION

Electrochemical measurements have indicated that the composition of the bone cement can influence a metal's response to localized corrosion. For 316L stainless steel and CoCrMo it can be seen that when a metal is combined with antibiotic bone cement, an increase susceptibility to localized corrosion can occur.

Figure 17

SEM Image of corrosion product within the CoCrMo and AB_3 bone cement crevice.

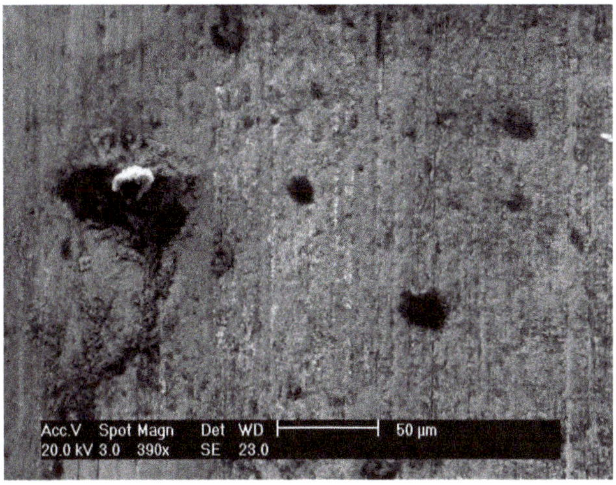

Figure 18

E_b of 316L with different additions.

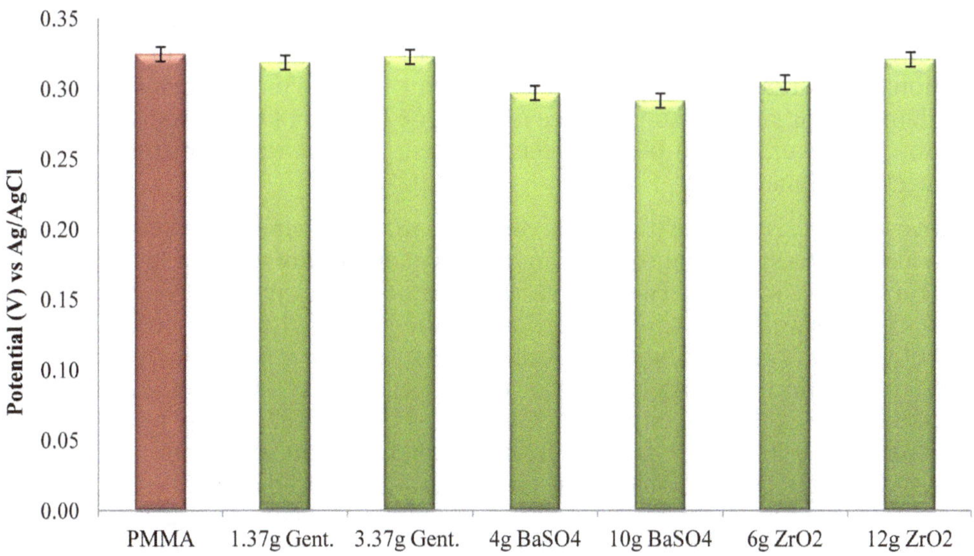

The breakdown potential of a material has been shown to be a quantitative method of accessing a materials resistance to loss of passivity due to pit initiation. Electrochemical measurements have indicated that for both materials, the presence of antibiotic in the bone cement can increase a material's susceptibility to localized crevice corrosion. It was found that the NA_1 bone cement had an increased resistance to localized crevice corrosion whilst the AB_2 bone cement was identified as the most susceptible to localized corrosion.

Repassivation potential measurements also provided interesting findings for the CoCrMo samples. A higher repassivation potential for CoCrMo samples when combined with NA_1 bone cement were noted, compared to samples combined with other bone

Figure 19

ΔE values for CoCrMo Alloy.

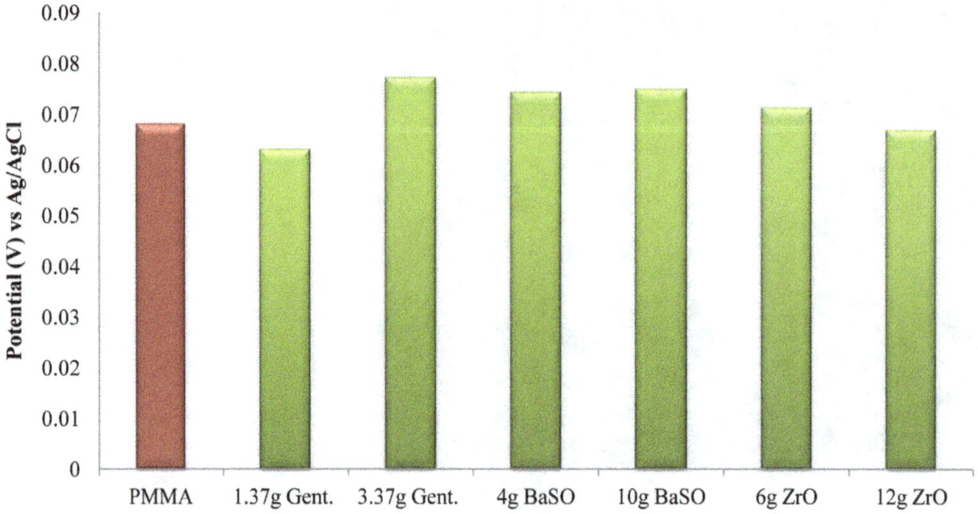

cements. It is considered the presence and concentration of different sulphate ions within the crevice could play a role in a materials susceptibility to localized corrosion. The presence of sulphate ions is known to affect the corrosion characteristics of a material, being associated with shifting the breakdown potential in the cathodic direction and increasing current density indicating that the presence of sulphate ions will inhibit pit initiation. The presence of chloride ions has been associated with pit imitation. However, once a pit has been initiated, pit growth dominates due to the presences of sulphate ions.[11, 12]

Negative hysteresis was also present on the potentiodynamic curves for both the 316L and CoCrMo samples; however, an increased amount of negative hysteresis was noted for the 316L samples. The hysteresis is created by the current density difference between the forward and reverse portions of the scan at the same potential. It is a result of the disruption of the passivation chemistry of the surface by the increase in potential and reflects the ease with which that passivation is restored as the potential is decreased towards the free corrosion potential.[13] Polarization to more noble potential causes a decrease in passivity, usually by initiation of localized corrosion, so that when the same potential reached on the reverse scan, the measured current emanates from a surface that is less passive.[13] In our case, this phenomenon is usually a reflection of a propensity for localized crevice corrosion to occur. Again, it can be seen from electrochemical analysis that bone cements containing antibiotic bone cements can increase a metals susceptibility to localized corrosion to occur.

Surface analysis of the specimens combined with commercially-available antibiotic cement further complemented the electrochemical analysis. Optical microscope observations demonstrated that crevice corrosion had occurred on all of the samples. SEM analysis demonstrated that a layer had been deposited on the surface of the 316L samples due to the corrosion process. Areas of localized pitting were also observed within the crevice area of the samples. For the 316L stainless steel samples, areas of pitting were macroscopically visible. SEM analysis indicated that intergranular corrosion had occurred within the crevice of the 316L specimens. Although electrochemical corrosion had occurred on the CoCrMo sample the extent of corrosion was not as great compared to the 316L stainless steel samples. SEM images indicate that small areas of pitting and localized regions of blackening had occurred on the CoCrMo surface.

As well as producing a novel test method capable of assessing and ranking a material in terms of its resistance to crevice corrosion when combined with different PMMA bone cements, the effects of different additives could be investigated whilst creating consistent and repeatable findings. The results presented in this study are from a simple design of experiments consisting of few variables, none the less the results obtained allow us to further our knowledge of how different constituents affect the localized corrosion mechanisms occurring at the stem-cement interface.

The results in this study have shown that for CoCrMo, the addition of radiopaque agents and antibiotic were seen to have no significant effect on the initiation mechanisms of localized crevice corrosion. However, the amount of propagation was seen to vary with the addition of radiopaque agents. Conversely, for the 316L samples it was found that the addition of such additives affected the initiation mechanisms, with the addition of barium sulphate reducing passivity the most when compared to a plain PMMA base cement. One hypothesis is that the introduction of radiopaque and antibiotic agents into the PMMA bone cement may cause favorable conditions for the initiation and propagation of electrochemical corrosion. It has long been established that the introduction of chloride and sulphate ions can increase a materials susceptibility to localized corrosion, with extensive research detailing the effects of these ions on the initiation and propagation mechanisms of localized corrosion. Studies have shown that chloride ions can be linked with the initiation stages of crevice corrosion, whilst sulphate ions have been shown to inhibit initiation, but promote propagation once the initiation has occurred.[11, 12] Antibiotics are commonly used in sulphate form to ensure their solubility *in vivo*. Antibiotics have been shown to leach out of the bone cement over time from exposed surfaces and pores.[7] It is thought that this leaching out of antibiotics from the PMMA bone cement may result in an addition of sulphate ions within the crevice, creating conditions favorable of crevice corrosion. Barium sulphate is also extensively used as a radiopaque agent to enable the bone cement to be visible under radiographs, which may add to the sulphate ion levels within the crevice though a similar leaching mechanism.

CONCLUSION

In conclusion, this study has demonstrated that the addition of antibiotics and radiopaque agents can affect the crevice corrosion mechanisms of commonly used orthopaedic materials. The results from this study provide useful information of how the use of PMMA bone cements can affect the localized degradation of commonly used biomaterials. For 316L stainless steel, this study has demonstrated that the addition of antibiotics and radiopaque agents can affect the initiation and propagation mechanisms of crevice corrosion, with the addition of barium sulphate having a predominant effect when compared with base PMMA cement. Benchmark testing on the CoCrMo samples indicated that the type of cement can affect the initiation and propagation mechanisms. However further cement variation studies are required to fully understand how each component affects the crevice corrosion mechanism and to establish if any interactions exist between each cement component. Studies into the effects of galvanic coupling, surface roughness and dynamic loading also need to be conducted to fully understand the role crevice corrosion plays in the overall degradation of cemented stems.

REFERENCES

1. Jacobs J., Gilbert J., Urban R. Current concepts review - Corrosion of metal orthopaedic implants. *The Journal of Bone and Joint Surgery* 1998;80:268-282.
2. Donell S., Darrah C., Nolan J., Wimhurst J., Toms A., Barker T., Case C., Tucker J. Early failure of the Ultima metal - on - metal total hip replacement in the presence of normal plain radiographs. *Journal of bone and joint surgery* 2010;92:1501-1508.
3. Bolland DC B., Langston D., Millington J., Arden N., Latham J. High Failure rates with a large-diameter hybrid metal-on-metal total hip replacement. *The Journal of Bone and Joint Surgery* 2011;93:608-615.
4. Willert H., Broback L., Buchhorn G., Jemsen P., Koster G., Lang I., Ochsner P., Schenk R. Crevice corrosion of cemented titanium alloy stems in total hip replacements. *Clin Orthop Relat Res* 1996;333:333-351.
5. Thomas S., Shukla D., Latham P. Corrosion of cemented titanium femoral stems. *Journal of bone and joint surgery* 2004;86:974-978.
6. Lautenschlager E., Marshall G., Marks K., Schwartz J., Nelson C. Mechanical strength of acrylic bone cements impregnated with antibiotics. *Journal of Biomedical Materials Research* 1976;10:837-845.
7. van de Belt H., Neut D., Uges D., Schenk W., van Horn J., van der Mei H., Busscher H. Surface roughness, porosity and wettability of gentamicin-loaded bone cements and their antibiotic release. *Biomaterials* 2000;21:1981-1987.
8. Oldfeild J., Sutton W. Crevice Corrosion of Stainless Steel I - A Mathematical Model. *Corrosion journal* 1978;13:13-22.
9. ASTM International ASTM F746-09 (2009) Standard test method for pitting or crevice corrosion of metallic surgical implant materials. In: 2009.
10. Oldfield JW, Sutton WH Crevice Corrosion of Stainless Steels. EROCOR '77, Eur Congr on Met Corros, 92nd Event of the Eur Fed of Corros 1977:239-246.
11. Lee W., Pyun S. Effects of sulphate ion additives on the pitting corrosion of pure aluminium in 0.01M NaCl solution. *Electrochemical Acta* 200;25:501.
12. Flis J., Kowalczyk K. *Journal of Applied Electrochemistry* 1995;25:501.
13. Silverman D. Tutorial on Cyclic Potentiodynamic Polarization Technique. Corrosion 98 1998.

Paper Number:
C2012-01591

Flow Assisted Corrosion Effects on Nitinol for Biomedical Applications

Elizabeth Trillo
Environmental Performance of Materials

Carl Popelar
Environmental Performance of Materials

James Dante
Environmental Performance of Materials

Abstract

Nitinol as a biomedical alloy has become an ideal material for use as self-expanding stents, grafts and other support systems due to its excellent superelasticity, biocompatibility and corrosion resistance. In terms of corrosion resistance, many studies have focused on the effects of surface treatments, oxide thickness, strain and presence of contaminants. However, in addition to these issues, a cardiovascular stent will also see the effect of pulsatile flow of blood through the artery. Thus, this work assessed the effects of fluid flow on the corrosion behavior of a super elastic Nitinol alloy. Electrochemical potentials were obtained on the Nitinol material while under flow conditions with a simulated body fluid. The electrochemical potential drifted positive after one week of continuous monitoring and ranged between --37 to 60 mV. Lower pH testing increased the overall corrosion potential. Post-test surface appearance was documented by Scanning Electron Microscopy (SEM). The flow conditions did not result in appreciable breakdown of the oxide layer.

Keywords: Flow assisted corrosion, Nitinol, biomaterial

INTRODUCTION

Metallic stents are typically hollow cylindrical tubes that control the blood flow in damaged vessels. Their function is to repair the vessel during artery obstruction during plaque build-up or from vascular rupture. Stent materials have been typically stainless steel or nickel-titanium alloys (Nitinol). The later material has been favored due to its shape memory and superelastic properties allowing stent devices to be placed in numerous locations in the body.[1-3] For such devices, the long term corrosion resistance and biocompatibility are of great interest.

Nitinol has a very adherent oxide layer (TiO_2 and NiO)[4] which has provided some corrosion resistance in biological fluid environments. The corrosion or breakdown of this layer, however, is of critical importance because of the toxic and carcinogenic effects of nickel in the human body.[5-8] Nickel ion dissolution and release is a potential problem which is largely an effect of the surface stability and chemistry.

Nitinol is known to be highly dependent on the surface condition and geometry of the component.[9] Removing the surface roughness by electropolishing will assist in blood biocompatibility and minimize blood clotting. Breakdown potentials were also lower and test results were also more reproducible for mechanically polished samples than unpolished Nitinol wires exposed to simulated body fluids.[10] Much attention has been placed in comparing different surface conditions of Nitinol stents in terms of corrosion resistance and biocompatibility to determine the optimum approach.[11-12] The corrosion resistance was higher when the oxide layer was mainly composed of TiO_2.[13-14] However, there is little or no attention to the effect of blood flow on the corrosion resistance of metallic stents, especially long term effects.

To address this gap, this work evaluates the open circuit potentials of Nitinol wire material over time in a simulated biological fluid while under flow conditions. Comparisons are made after one week exposures. The effects of lower pH conditions are also evaluated. Cyclic potentiodynamic polarization testing was performed after the week-long exposure to determine the overall and localized corrosion behavior. The surface characteristics were analyzed by Scanning Electron Microscopy (SEM).

EXPERIMENTAL PROCEDURE

Material

The Nitinol material utilized for this program was commercially available SE 08 (superelastic) wire. It had a nominal diameter of 0.3 mm. The material was nearly equiatomic Nickel (51%) and Titanium (49%). The wire was received with an etched surface condition. The surface oxide was measured to be 167 nm. No further processing was performed on the sires prior to testing.

Open Circuit Potential Monitoring

A length section of wire was used for open circuit potential monitoring. The wire was wound on a Teflon mandrel placed into a 1-L glass cell. There was approximately 1.5 in. of wire exposed to the solution after wrapping. Testing was performed on a rotating cylinder electrode (RCE) assembly to determine the flow effects on the wire. The rotational speed was selected to simulate the flow rate on a coronary artery (11.3 cm/s) without pulsatile effects. Phosphate Buffered Saline Solution at a pH of 7.4 was utilized as the test medium along with a saturated calomel electrode (SCE) as a reference electrode and platinum mesh for a counter electrode (see Figure 1). Testing was performed in duplicate at 37°C under a nitrogen purge. The open circuit potential was measured continuously for 7 days. A second series of tests were also performed with a PBS solution adjusted to a pH of 5.5. This was to simulate the low pH in areas where there are infected tissues. Scanning Electron Microscopy (SEM) was performed on the test samples after open circuit testing to determine if there were any flow effects on the surface of the samples.

Cyclic Potentiodynamic Polarization Testing

Cyclic Potentiodynamic Polarization testing was performed using both test solutions. Testing was performed in accordance with ASTM F2129. The SCE and platinum mesh were used as a reference and counter electrodes, respectively. The polarization test started at 50 mV below the OCP at a scan rate of 0.167 mV/sec. The scan was reversed at 900 mV back to the open circuit potential.

RESULTS

Open Circuit Potential

The open circuit measurements over time for the Nitinol wire tested in the PBS solution (pH 7.4) are presented in Figure 2. Duplicate tests were performed. Both tests showed the same behavior, although they are displaced slightly from one another. After 1 hour

Figure 1

Photograph of RCE electrochemical cell for open circuit measurements.

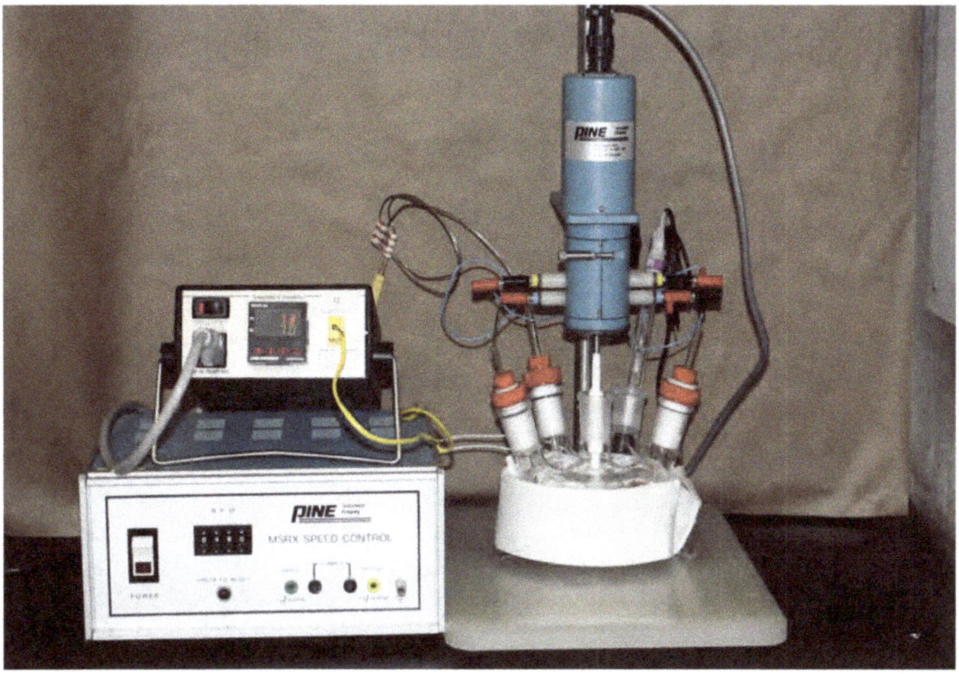

Figure 2

Open Circuit Potential vs. Time for Nitinol wire in PBS solution under flow conditions.

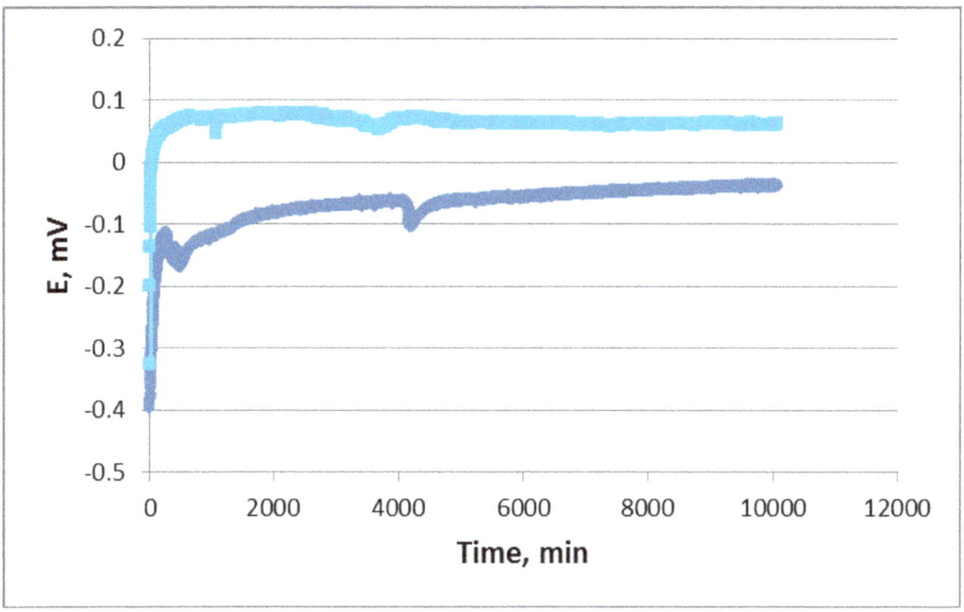

Figure 3

Open Circuit Potential vs. Time for Nitinol wire in a low pH PBS solution under flow conditions.

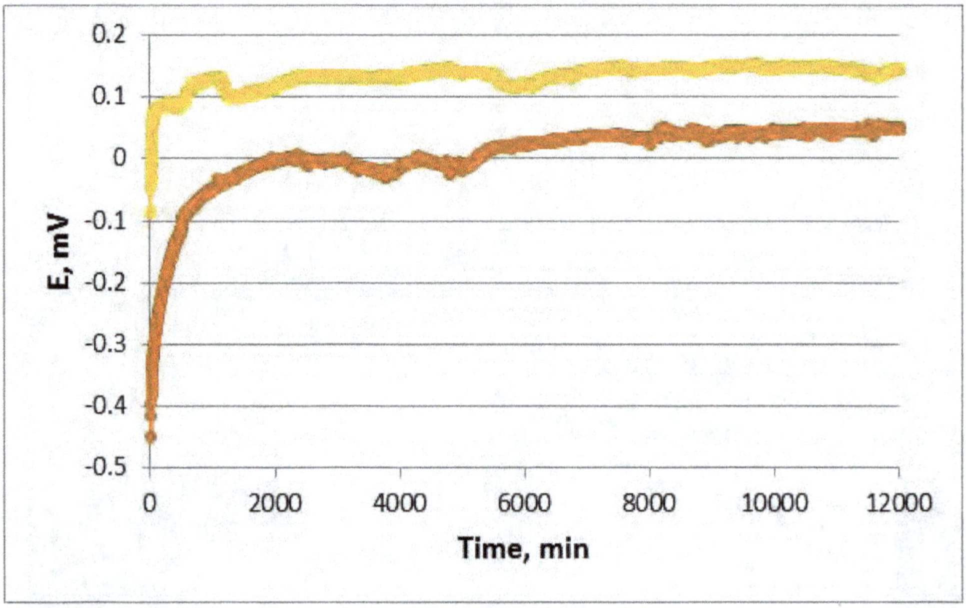

the open circuit potentials were -226 mV and 21 mV for the two wire samples tested. After 1 day the potentials were -97 mV and 74 mV, and after seven days of flow drift to valves of -37 mV and 60 mV. Table 1 documents these changes.

The results for the lower pH testing are seen in Figure 3. There is a small difference in potential between the duplicate tests, however, both samples did show the same behavior. After one hour testing under flow conditions, the open circuit potentials were -293 and 75 mV. After one day of flow testing the potentials increased to 22 and 104 mV and after 7 days testing the potentials increased to values of 44 and 150 mV.

The SEM analysis performed on an untested sample and samples after open circuit monitoring are seen in Figures 4 through 6. The samples did have some surface roughness prior to testing. After testing for 7 days, there was no evidence of general or localized corrosion. The samples essentially looked the same before and after testing.

TABLE 1

Open Circuit Potentials for Nitinol in PBS Solution with Flow.

Sample	1 Hour, mV	24 Hours, mV	7 Days, mV
Sample 1 / PBS	-226	-97	-37
Sample 2 / PBS	21	74	60
Sample 1 / PBS at 5.5 pH	-293	22	44
Sample 2 / PBS at 5.5 pH	75	104	150

Figure 4

SEM micrographs of Nitinol wire prior to testing a) 250x and b) 1000x.

a

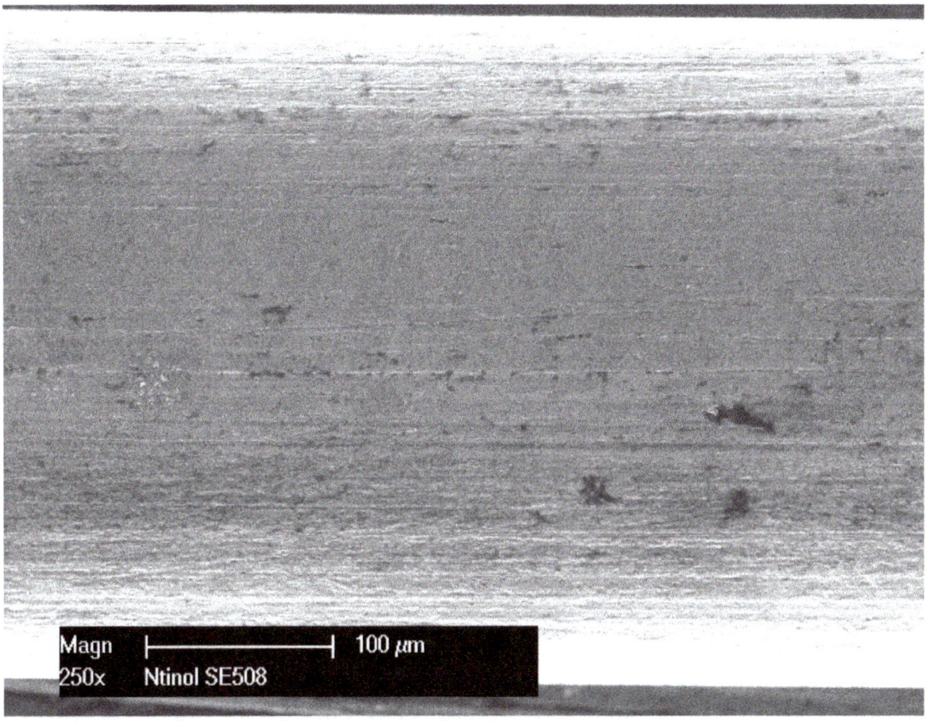

b

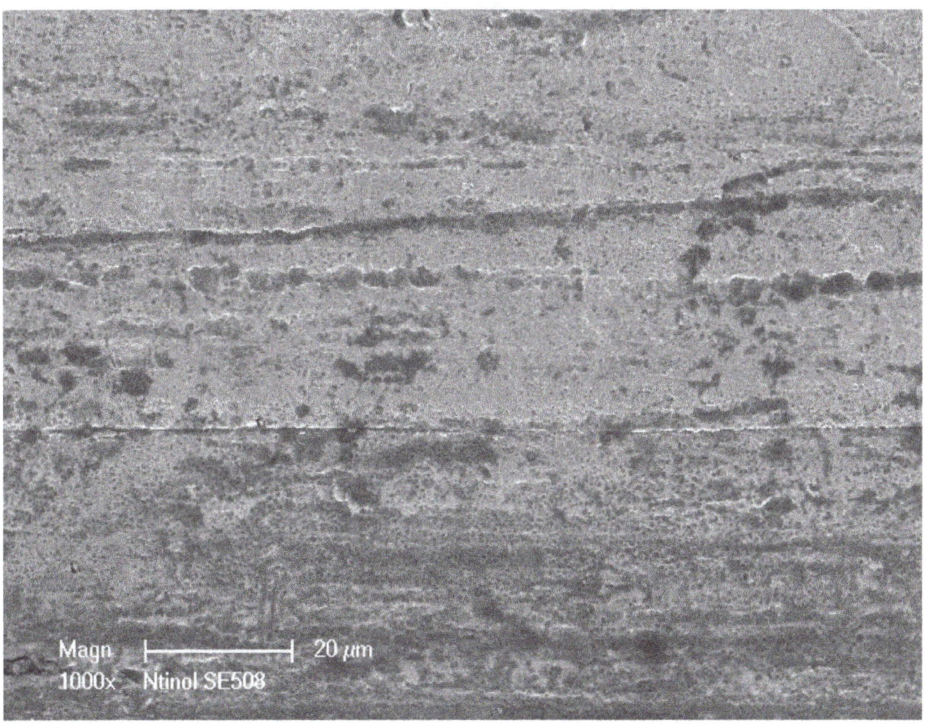

No cracking of the oxide layer was also observed either. It should be noted that the samples were observed on a mandrel inside the SEM such that it would keep the same radius of bend as was tested during the open circuit potential testing for 7 days.

Cyclic Potentiodynamic Polarization

Figures 7 and 8 present the cyclic potentiodynamic polarization scans performed on a section of Nitinol wire exposed to a PBS solution (pH 7.4) and a PBS solution with a 5.5 pH. The open circuit potentials were -317 mV and -200 mV for the PBS solution and low pH solution, respectively. Both scans show a passive region approximately 10^{-8} A/cm^2 with slight disruptions on the passive portion of the scan. The lower pH scan did show many more disruptions on the passive region than the PBS solution with pH 7.4. The pitting potential was 329 mV and 290 mV for the PBS and low pH solutions, respectively.

DISCUSSION

The potential monitoring performed in this study showed that a rapid increase in corrosion potential occurs for the first hour of continuous measurement under flow conditions. After one hour of testing, the open circuit values of both solutions were between -293 and 75 mV and were comparable to those that have been reported in the literature [16, 17]. The open circuit potential then slowly increased for the seven day test duration. This occurred for both samples with the PBS solution at 7.4 and 5.5 pH. Table 1 shows that the change in potential between the 1 hour and 24 hour exposures. For the PBS solution under flow conditions, this change is in the range of 53 to 129 mV and in the range of 29 and 315 mV for the lower pH test solution. After 24 hours, the potential still increased but at a much slower rate. The potential increase between the 24 hour and 7 day measurements for the PBS solution was 14 and 30 mV. The lower pH test solution had potentials readings and between 22 to 46 mV.

It should be noted that there was no major difference in open circuit potentials between the flow testing at PBS solution with 7.4 pH and the 5.5 pH. After 1 hour all values were in the range as was reported before. The cyclic polarization scans also had an open circuit potential in the range as seen above. In addition, the pitting potentials were also the same for both test solutions. The passive currents, although were the same current density, had many more disruptions on the passive region with the lower pH solution than with the pH 7.4 solution.

This research shows that flow assisted corrosion effects of physiological fluids did not appreciably change the corrosion behavior of the Nitinol wire. However, this study focused only on one diameter of wire with one thickness of oxide layer. Nitinol wires that have different sizes and/or are processed differently may have different results.

CONCLUSIONS

This study looked at the flow assisted corrosion effects of fluid flow on Nitinol material. Based on the electrochemical testing performed, the following observations were made:

Figure 5

SEM micrographs of Nitinol wire after 7 day open circuit testing in a PBS Solution a) 250x and b) 1000x.

a

b

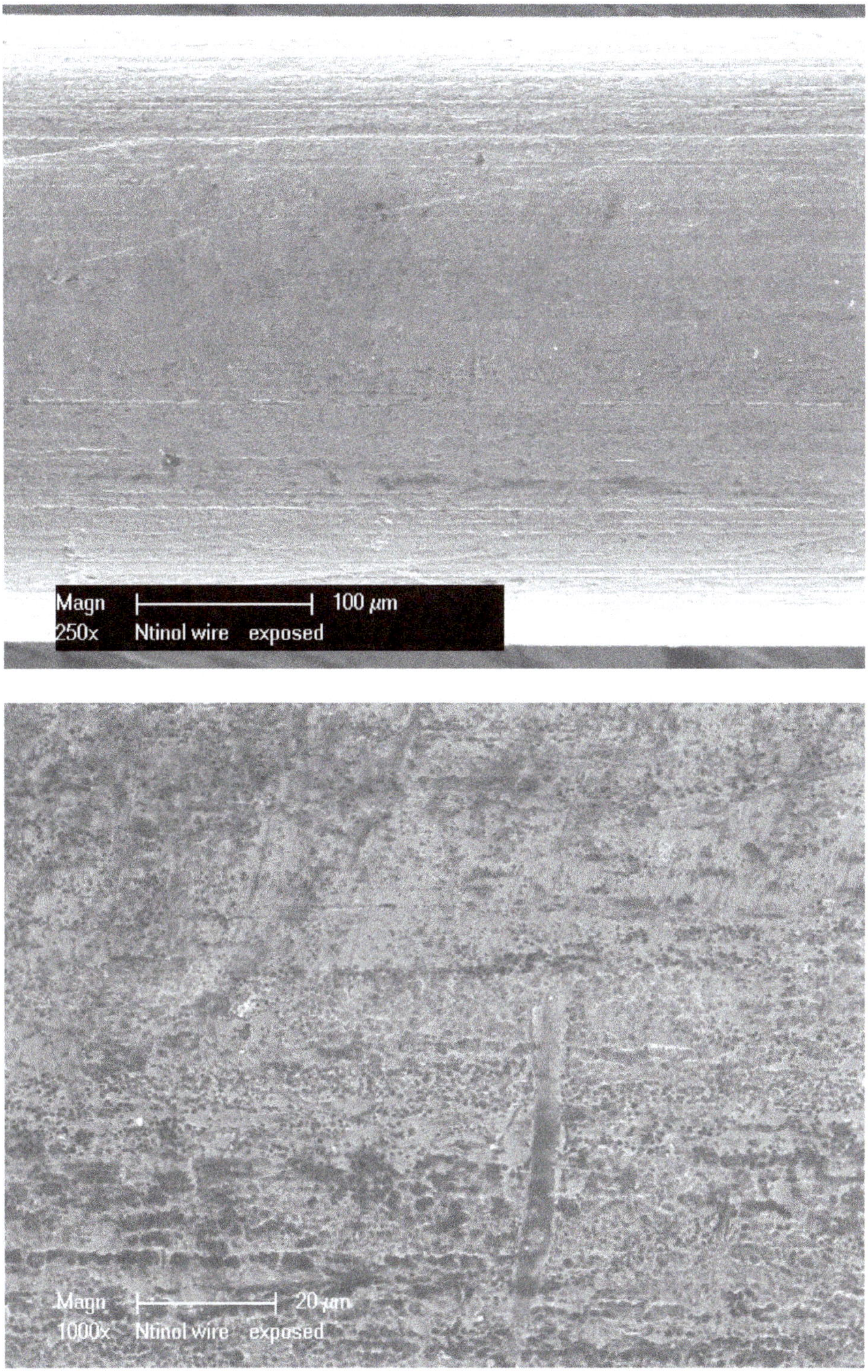

Figure 6

SEM micrographs of Nitinol wire after 7 day open circuit testing in a PBS solution with Low pH a) 250x and b) 1000x.

a

b

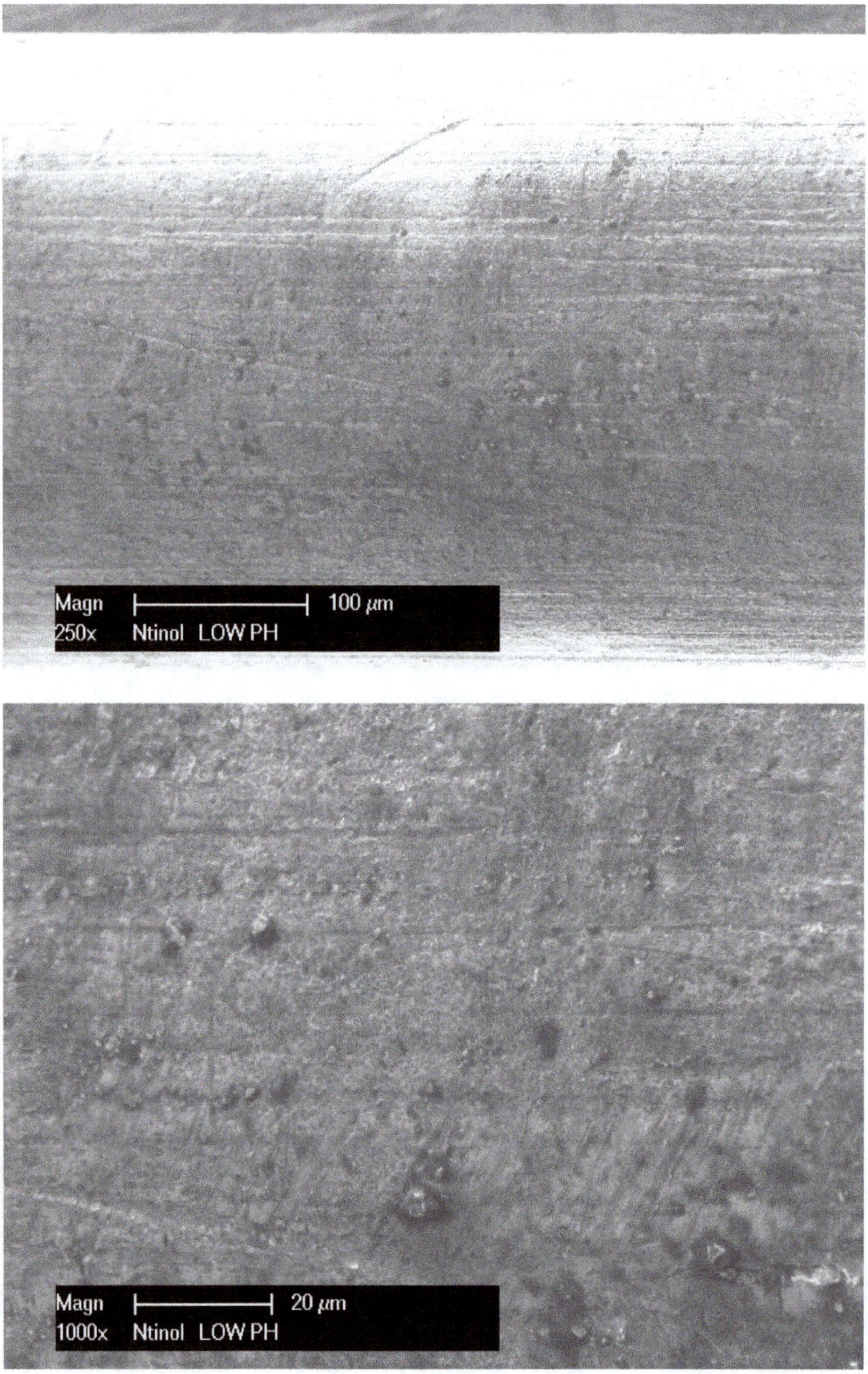

Figure 7

Cyclic Polarization Scan for a Nitinol wire in a PBS solution at pH 7.4 (without rotation).

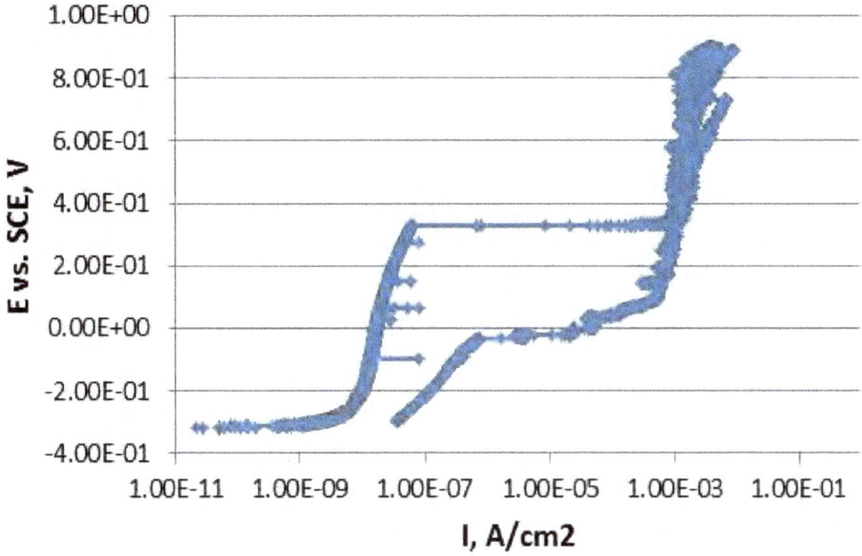

Figure 8

Cyclic Polarization Scan for a Nitinol wire in a PBS solution at pH 5.5 (without rotation).

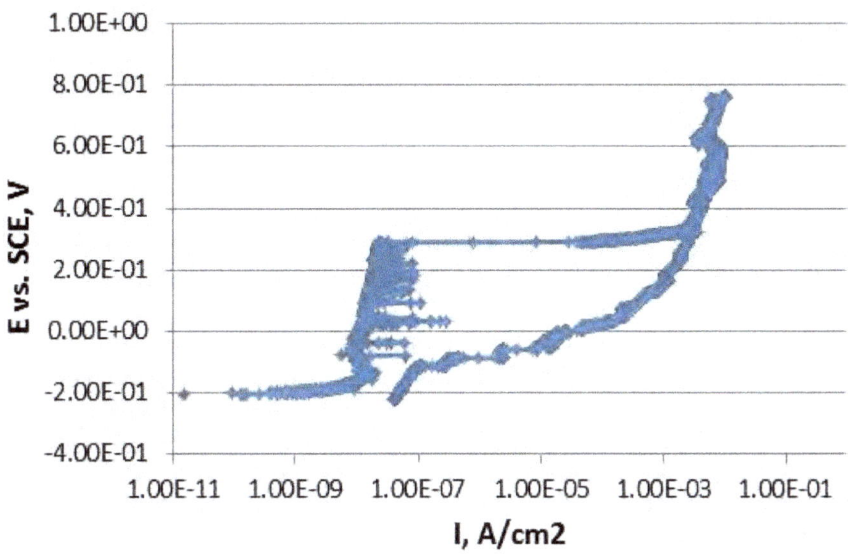

- Open circuit monitoring of Nitinol wire in PBS under flow conditions revealed a rapid increase in the corrosion potential for the first hour of continuous measurement. The open circuit potentials were in the range as reported by previous researchers.
- The open circuit potentials increased between the 1 hour and 24 hour measurements. The potential change was in the range of 53 to 129 mV for the PBS solution. The potential change was in the range of 29 and 315 mV for the lower pH test solution.
- The potential also increased between the 24 hour and the 7 day measurements, but at a much slower rate. The potential increase between the 24 hour and 7 day measurements for the PBS solution was 14 and 30 mV. The lower pH test solution had potentials readings and between 22 to 46 mV.
- The SEM analysis showed that there were no visible microstructural changes in the surface oxide layer after flow testing for 7 days compared to Nitinol wire examined prior to testing.
- The cyclic polarization scans showed that both the 7.4 pH and 5.5 pH test solutions had open circuit potentials that were within the reported range. The pitting potentials were also the same for both test solutions. The passive current densities were approximately the same for both solutions, however, there were much more disturbances with the lower pH solution.
- The flow of physiological fluid did not seem to greatly affect the corrosion behavior of Nitinol wire. However, other wire sizes and manufacturing may present different results.

REFERENCES

1. Funakubo H., Shape Memory Alloys, *Cordon and Breach Science Publishers*, 1984.
2. Duerig T., Pelton A. and Stoeckel D., "The utility of Superelasticity in Medicine", *Biomed. Mater. Eng*, 6, pp. 255-266, 1996.
3. Stoeckel D., "Nitinol Medical Devices and Implants", *Min Invas Ther Allied Technol*, 9, pp. 81-89, 2000.
4. Buehler WJ, Gilfrich JV, Wiley RC., "Effect of Low-Temperature Phase Changes on the Mechanical Properties of Alloys Near Composition NiTi", *J. Appl Phys*, 34(5), pp. 1475-1477, 1963.
5. McKay GC, Mcnair R, MacDonald C, Grant MH., "Interactions of Orthopaedic Metals with an Immortalised Rat Osteoblast Cell Line", *Biomaterials*, 17, pp. 1339-1344, 1996.
6. Goyer R., "Toxic Effect of Metals", *Cassarett and Doull's Toxicology*, Klassen C., Amdun M. and Doul J., eds, Macmillan, New York, pp. 582-635, 1986.
7. Hayes R., "The Carcinogenicity of Metals in Human", *Cancer Causes and Control*, 8, pp. 321-327, 1997.
8. Oller A. and Costa M., "Carcinoginicity Assessment of Selected Nickel Compounds", *Toxicol. Appl. Parmac.*, 143, pp. 152-166, 1997.
9. Shabalovskaya S., Rondelli G., Itin V. and Anderegg J., "Surface and Corrosion Aspects of NiTi Alloys", Third Int. Conf. Shape Memory and Superelastic Technologies, Pacific Grove, CA, May 2000.
10. Carroll WM and Kelly M.J., "Corrosion Behavior of Nitinol Wires in Body Fluid Environments", pp. 1123-1130, 2003.

11. Trigwell S., et al, "Effects of Surface Treatment on the Surface Chemistry of NiTi Alloy for Biomedical Applications", *Surf. Interface Anal*, 26, pp. 483-489, 1998.
12. Chan C-M. Trigwell S. , and Duerig T., "Oxidation of an NiTi Alloy", *Surf Interface Anal*, 15, pp. 349-354, 1990.
13. Wever D.J., Veldhuizen AG, de Vries J., Busscher HJ, Uges D.R.. and van Horn JR, "Electrochemical and Surface Characterization of a Nickel-Titanium Alloy", *Biomaterials*, 19, pp. 761-769, 1998.
14. Venugopalan R. and Trepanier C., "Assessing the Corrosion Behavior of Nitinol for Minimally Invasive Device Design", *Min Invas Ther Allied Technol*, 9(2), pp. 67-73, 2000.
15. Warner C.P., "The Effect of Exposure on Simulated Body Fluids on Breakdown Potentials", *Journal of Mat. Eng. And Performance*, 18, pp. 754-759, 2009.
16. Eiselstein L.E., Steffey D., Nissan A., Corlett N., Dugnani R., Kus E. and Steward S.G., "Acceptance Criteria for Corrosion Resistance of Medical Devices: Statistical Analysis of Nitinol Pitting in In Vivo Environments", *Journal of Mat. Eng And Performance*, 18, pp. 768-780, 2009.
17. Pound B.G., "Susceptibility of Nitinol to Localized Corrosion", *J. of Biomed. Mater. Res. A*, 77 (1), pp. 185-191, 2006.

Paper Number:
C2023-19522

Development of New Grades of Titanium-Based Metal Glasses for Dental Applications

Dr. Benoît Ter-Ovanessian
INSA Lyon / MATEIS

Abstract

Ti-based metallic glasses, dedicated to biomedical applications, were first designed by adding large amounts of Ni, Be or Cu to achieve the highest possible glass-forming ability. It is straightforward that those elements are not fully compatible with biomedical applications such as biocompatibility or long-life implants. This work, following an approach based on material design by corrosion performance, proposes different new compositions of Ti-based metallic glasses suitable for dental applications. The corrosion behavior of the new grades was analyzed by electrochemical tests according to standard ISO 10271, for dentistry applications. Corrosion performance was also analyzed through immersion tests for a period of 4 weeks at 37°C. The role of Ti, Zr, Cu and Si contents on the pitting behavior is discussed.

Keywords: Corrosion resistant alloys, Titanium alloys, amorphous alloys, biomedical, pitting corrosion

INTRODUCTION

Nowadays, titanium-based alloys are commonly used in biomedical applications as, for example, materials for dental implants or hip replacements. Their good corrosion resistance, biocompatibility and high mechanical properties for a relative weight make them good candidates[1–3]. However, improvements in the design of these alloys for biomedical applications need to be made. Firstly, some of the alloys currently in use have elements such as Al or V which are suspected to be toxic[4]. Secondly, the elasticity moduli of current materials are too high compared to that of bone. Stress shielding phenomena can therefore occur, sometimes leading to the loss of the prosthesis [5]. Finally, in the context of the development of less invasive surgery, the mechanical properties of these alloys are not sufficient to manufacture smaller implants or prostheses resistant to complex stresses.

Two main paths for the development of titanium alloys for biomedical applications are currently being explored: the design of low modulus titanium alloys (with an emphasis on the beta phase)[6–8] and the design of bulk metallic glass (BMG)[9–12]. The use of BMG is of particular interest in the dental field as it would allow the miniaturization of implants[13,14]. The latter would be compatible with different jaw morphologies and would limit some aesthetic concerns. Furthermore, the corrosion behavior is generally improved for BMG in comparison with their crystalline counterpart due to the lack of defects (grain boundaries, second phases...).

The possibilities in terms of the composition of metallic glasses are tremendous[15]. However, some of these materials can only be obtained in small dimensions or even as thin films. Thus, in our case, it is necessary to develop compositions that will be the most efficient according to: (i) their amorphization potential generally described by the glass forming ability (GFA) or the critical diameter (maximal diameter for which the material is fully amorphous), (ii) their high mechanical properties, (iii) their long-term biocompatibility, (iv) their resistance to corrosion and to mechanically assisted corrosion. Many design studies of these materials focus on the first three items and only evaluate the corrosion behavior afterwards. Furthermore, improvement in one of these characteristics is often at the expense of another. As a result, the deployment of BMG in the medical field remains anecdotal compared to their potential.

In this study, based on a literature survey and a preliminary study of a widely studied grade[10,11], the chemical and microstructural weaknesses have been identified in order to propose new grades with better corrosion performance. Firstly, the TiZrCuPd system was studied to discuss the role of transition elements in metallic glasses and the interest of their substitution. Then, TiZrSiGeBSn alloys were studied in order to highlight the role of the Ti/Zr ratio on the sensitivity to localized corrosion. All these materials were tested in a naturally aerated solution of 0.9 wt% NaCl with a pH= 7 ± 0.1 and at 37°C according to standard ISO 10271, for dentistry applications[16].

EXPERIMENTAL PROCEDURE

Material Processing Routes

Master alloys, with targeted compositions Ti40Zr10Cu36Pd14, Ti40Zr10Cu34Pd14Sn2, Ti40Zr10Cu33Pd14Sn2Si1, Ti50Zr30Si8Ge7B3Sn2, Ti50Zr30Si5Ge5B5Sn5, Ti40Zr40Si8Ge7B3Sn2, and Ti40Zr40Si5Ge5B5Sn5 (at. %), were prepared by arc melting the pure elements (purities above 99.9%). Rods with a diameter of 5 mm for Ti40Zr10Cu36Pd14, Ti40Zr10Cu34Pd14Sn2 and Ti40Zr10Cu33Pd14Sn2Si1 were prepared using a tilt copper mold-casting apparatus in a high purity argon atmosphere. The four other alloys were melt-spun using a melt spinner device with a rotating copper

Table 1

Tested materials' atomic composition and assigned names.

Material label	Ti (%at.)	Zr (%at.)	Cu (%at.)	Pd (%at.)	Sn (%at.)	Si (%at.)	B (%at.)	Ge (%at.)
TiZrCuPd*	40	10	36	14	-	-	-	-
TiZrCuPdSn*	40	10	34	14	2	-	-	-
TiZrCuPdSnSi*	40	10	33	14	2	1	-	-
Ti50Zr30-Si8-Sn2	50	30	-	-	2	8	3	7
Ti50Zr30-Si5-Sn5	50	30	-	-	5	5	5	5
Ti40Zr40-Si8-Sn2	40	40	-	-	2	8	3	7
Ti40Zr40-Si5-Sn5	40	40	-	-	5	5	5	5

* Material obtained in rod form while the other were ribbons

wheel of 26 mm after ingot homogenization. The last test materials were processed in ribbon form to facilitate the production of a large number of samples to ensure reproducibility of the tests.

The composition of all the material was controlled by Energy-Dispersive X-Ray spectroscopy (EDX) on a Scanning Electron Microscope (SEM) at an acceleration voltage of 15 keV. Table 1 reported the composition of the tested materials and their label furtherly used.

Structural Characterization

Before performing the corrosion behavior studies, the glassy structure of obtained materials was checked. The amorphous nature of all the samples after processing was estimated by X-Ray Diffraction (XRD) analysis, using Co-Kα radiation. Glass transition temperature (Tg) and crystallization temperature (Tx) were characterized by Differential Scanning Calorimetry (DSC) at a heating rate of 20 K/min under high purity dry nitrogen at a flow rate of 20 mL/min. In the present study, all tested materials were assumed amorphous at the XRD scale. Extensive characterization by TEM would be required to confirm this result.

Corrosion Performance Characterization

Electrochemical Characterization

The corrosion behavior of the different materials was studied by electrochemical tests in a naturally aerated solution of NaCl at 0.9 wt% at a pH= 7 ± 0.1 and at 37°C (ISO 10271, for dentistry applications) [16]. The electrochemical measurements were performed with a potentiostat Reference 600 [1] in a three-electrode glass cell. The tested materials were used as working electrodes. A silver-silver chloride electrode (Ag/AgCl) and a graphite electrode were used as reference and counter electrodes, respectively. Rods samples were covered with a heat-shrinkable sheath, leaving only the tip of the cylinder in contact with the solution. Before the electrochemical measurements, the rod disc surface was ground down to #2400 using abrasive papers. For ribbons, the working surface was measured by optical microscopy before the test after delimiting the working area with blocking varnish.

As the materials presented in this study came from different collaborators and were initially dedicated to different studies, two different procedures were used for rods and ribbons:

- The Open Circuit Potential (OCP) of rods (TiZrCuPd, TiZrCuPdSn, TiZrCuPdSnSi) was monitored during 24 h. Electrochemical Impedance Spectroscopy measurements were conducted at 6 and 24 h at the reached open-circuit potential in the frequency range of $5x10^{-3}$ Hz to 10^5 Hz using an amplitude of 10 mV_{RMS} and 9 points per decade. Finally, a linear sweep voltammetry was performed with a scan rate of 0.166 mV/s from −0.2 to +1 V vs. Ag/AgCl.
- For ribbons (Ti50Zr30-Si8-Sn2, Ti50Zr30-Si5-Sn5, Ti40Zr40-Si8-Sn2, Ti40Zr40-Si5-Sn5), the OCP was monitored for 2 h to check the stabilization of the working electrode/electrolyte interface. Then cyclic polarization was performed with a

[1] Gamry instrument, 734 Louis Drive, Warminster, PA 18974, US

rate of 1 mV/s for forward and reverse scans. The forward scan started from -0.2 V vs. OCP and stopped at +2.5 V vs. SCE or when the current density reached $2mA/cm^2$. The reverse scan stopped at 0 V vs. OCP.

At least six tests were performed for each composition and electrolyte for statistical information. After the electrochemical test, the exposed surface was observed with SEM.

Passive Film Characterization

The passive film chemistry of the Ti-based glassy alloys was analyzed by an X-ray photoelectron spectrometer (XPS) with a monochromatic Al Kα source of 1486.6 eV and a beam-to-detector angle of 45° after 24 h immersed at 37°C in the 9% NaCl. The binding energy was calibrated using the carbon peak at 284.6 eV. The data were fitted with Shirley background and Gaussian Lorentzian line shape.

Immersion Tests

The tested material's ion release, mass loss, and pH changes over time were monitored through immersion tests. After ethanol cleaning, the samples were weighed and immersed for four weeks in NaCl at 0.9 wt% and at 37°C. The solution/area ratio used was 0.016 mm^{-1}. The flasks with each sample in different solutions were collocated in an incubator-shaker device at constant agitation of 50 RPM. Each week the pH was measured, and the solutions were changed for fresh ones. The ions released in the solutions were analyzed by ICP-MS. The ribbons were weighed at the end of the test, and the mass loss was reported.

RESULTS

The result section will be divided into two parts. The first one devoted to the study of the alloys TiZrCuPd, TiZrCuPdSn, TiZrCuPdSnSi aims to highlight the weak points of these grades. The second part is dedicated to the study of the Ti50Zr30-Si8-Sn2, Ti50Zr30-Si5-Sn5, Ti40Zr40-Si8-Sn2, Ti40Zr40-Si5-Sn5 alloys and aims at demonstrating the potentialities of these new compositions. Additional results on structural characterization and corrosion performance have been published elsewhere [17,18]. The structural characterization will not be discussed here. All the tested materials were detected as fully amorphous by XRD measurement.

Corrosion behavior of TiZrCuPd, TiZrCuPdSn, TiZrCuPdSnSi alloys

Role of the chemical composition and the casting defects on the corrosion behavior of TiZrCuPd

Figure 1a represents the polarization curves obtained after a 24h immersion in the saline solution for the metallic glass TiZrCuPd and for the titanium alloy (TA6V) which is currently the reference material for biomedical uses.

In the case of TA6V, a passive behavior is observed over a large potential range with a very low current density. For metallic glass, it is important to note that, compared to TA6V, the shape of the cathodic branch is different, the corrosion potential is slightly lower, the current density of the passive plateau is higher and a sudden increase in the current density (qualifying the breakdown of the passive film) is observed. Thus, metallic glass, although having a passive character, seems very sensitive to

Figure 1

Polarization curves obtained on TiZrCuPd and TA6V alloys after 24h of immersion 0,9%NaCl at 37°C with a scan rate of 0.166 mV/s (a) and localized corrosion details observed after an interrupted test on TiZrCuPd alloy (b).

(a) (b)

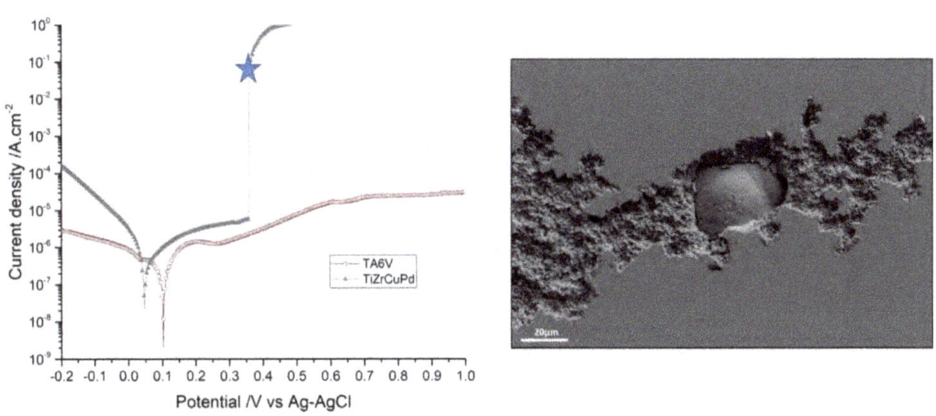

localized corrosion. Figure 1b shows a detail of the attacked surface after an interrupted polarization test at 0.1 A.cm^{-2}. The purpose of this interrupted test was to highlight the zones most likely to the initiation of localized corrosion. On this picture, a randomly distributed attack on the surface of the sample, and an attack that seems to be initiated at the vicinity of spherical crystalline defects are observed. This crystalline defect, also called spherulite, has already been reported in the literature [17,18]. It is a complex multi-phase precipitate with a core-shell structure. The precipitation and growth mechanisms of this casting defect are still not totally understood.

At this stage, it is important to note that:

- the crystalline defects thus revealed by the etching are not detected by XRD, indicating that this technique is not sufficient to quantify the amorphous nature of the metallic glasses. Scanning and transmission electron microscopy analyses are necessary to confirm the glassy state.
- the crystalline defects, and in particular the interface between the defect and the amorphous matrix are privileged sites for localized corrosion initiation [17,19].
- the composition of the amorphous matrix does not seem to be completely homogeneous, and some areas are more sensitive than others.

According to the literature, the susceptibility to localized corrosion of these grades is related to their high copper content and the process of formation of the passive film in a saline environment [17,20,21]. For both Ti and Zr bases, the passive film is formed by preferential oxidation of Ti or Zr, leading to an enrichment in Cu of the underlying metal. This enrichment could induce an auto-catalytic effect during the propagation of a localized corrosion defect. According to Flaviu *et al.*[20] the susceptibility of Zr-based BMG to pitting corrosion is directly attributable to the Cu content. In the work of Li *et al.*[22] different Zr-based alloys were studied. The authors then highlighted that the sensitivity to pitting corrosion was related to the nature of the transition element used. Cu induced more sensitivity than Co and Ni.

Figure 2

Polarization curves obtained on TiZrCuPdn, TiZrCuPdSn, TiZrCuPdSnSi and TA6V alloys after 24h of immersion 0,9%NaCl at 37°C with a scan rate of 0.166 mV/s.

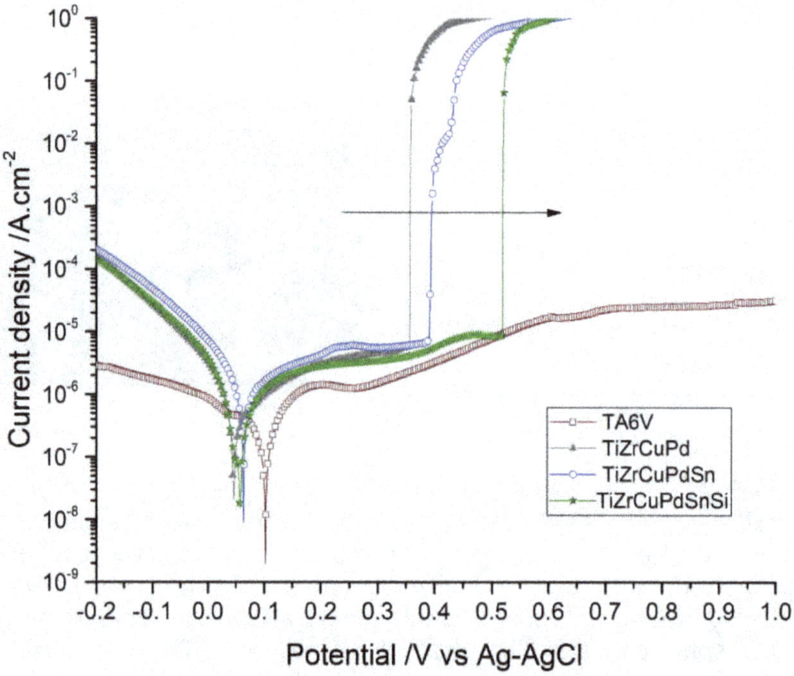

Thus, it is important to decrease the Cu content of these alloys, even if this element is a key element of amorphization. Indeed, this element is often used in BMG compositions because it ensures a high GFA. Indeed, Cu exhibits a significant atomic size mismatch with Ti or Zr and negative heats of mixing with the other alloying elements, insuring a glassy structure. However, for some BMG compositions and under specific casting conditions, a high amount of Cu in the alloy also prone the presence of crystal defects. This could be explained by an early precipitation in the melt linked to a heterogeneous chemical composition of the melt or the presence of oxide in it. It would result during solidification in these casting defects and zones more or less enriched in Cu in the amorphous matrix.

Thus, it is important to decrease the Cu content in these alloys in order to reduce their susceptibility to pitting corrosion but also to limit the presence of casting defects.

Effect of Substituting Cu by Sn and Si

In an attempt to maintain a high GFA, 2-3% at. Cu was substituted by Sn and Si. The polarization curves obtained for these two new alloys (under the same experimental conditions) are reported in Figure 2. The average values, obtained from 6 tests, of corrosion potential, passive current density, pitting potential are reported in Table 2. In agreement with what has been discussed previously, the range of passivity potential ($\eta_{pit} = E_{pit} - E_{corr}$) is wider as the Cu content decreases.

Figure 3

SEM observations of the exposed surface of TiZrCuPdn(a), TiZrCuPdSn (b), TiZrCuPdSn-Si(c) after the polarization test performed in 0,9%NaCl at 37°C.

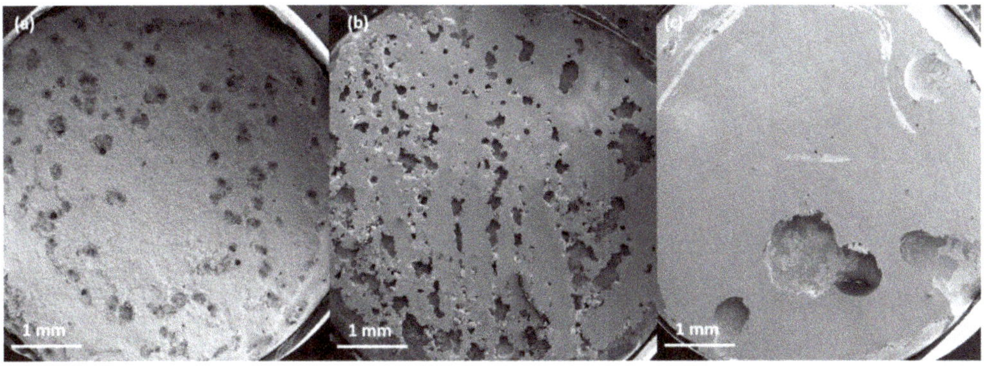

In addition, the study of the surfaces after the polarization tests indicates a different behavior between these three alloys (Figure 3). For the TiZrCuPd alloy (Figure 3a), as mentioned previously, the surface is very corroded. Deeper corrosion pits are observed at the crystalline defects. In the case of alloy TiZrCuPdSn (Figure 3b), the surface is less corroded. The presence of crystalline defects is also revealed by the corrosion in lesser quantities. The corrosion zones are less scattered on the surface. Finally, for the alloy TiZrCuPdSnSi (Figure 3b), the corroded surface is very different. There are only a few large and smooth attacked areas. For the latter alloy, no spherulite was detected.

This finding confirms the harmful character of a high Cu content in these metallic glasses, both for the structural quality of the glass and for its corrosion resistance. The substitution of Sn and Si has the effect of limiting the precipitation of casting defects, of making the chemical composition of the matrix more homogeneous and consequently of reducing the sensitivity to pitting corrosion. It is therefore important to develop new metallic glasses by limiting the Cu content or even excluding this element from the alloy.

Corrosion Behavior of the TiZrSiGeBSn Alloys

Electrochemical Characterization

The cyclic potentiodynamic curves obtained on the four different ribbons are shown in Figure 4. The obtained curves are representative of passive material in a chloride-containing solution. A passive plateau is observable in the anodic potential domain up to the sudden increase of current density related to pitting occurrence. The means

Table 2

Corrosion resistance indicators obtained from the polarization studies on TiZrCuPdn, TiZrCuPdSn, TiZrCuPdSnSi.

Sample	E_{corr} mV vs AgAgCl	I pass μA.cm^{-2}	E pit mV vs AgAgCl	η pit mV
TiZrCuPd	21 ± 71	3.97 ± 0.42	381 ± 66	360 ± 104
TiZrCuPdSn	29 ± 61	4.26 ± 0.67	410 ± 72	381 ± 113
TiZrCuPdSnSi	29 ± 10	3.31 ± 0.34	480 ± 54	451 ± 45

Figure 4

Polarization curves obtained on Ti50Zr30-Si8-Sn2, Ti50Zr30-Si5-Sn5, Ti40Zr40-Si8-Sn2, Ti40Zr40-Si5-Sn5 alloys after 2h of immersion 0,9%NaCl at 37°C with a scan rate of 1 mV/s.

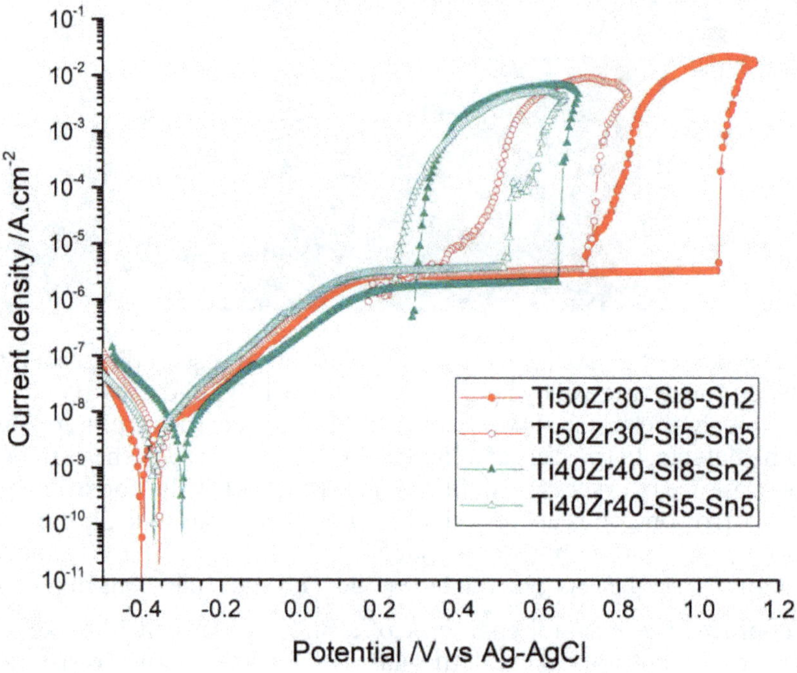

value of the corrosion potential (Ecorr), passivation current density (Ipass), pitting potential (Epit), and repassivation potential (Epp), determined by forward and reverse scan are resumed in Table 3. The passivation domain η_{pit} is also reported, indicating the resistance to stable pit initiation. The higher this value, the higher the resistance.

Table 3

Corrosion resistance indicators obtained from the polarization studies on Ti50Zr30-Si8-Sn2, Ti50Zr30-Si5-Sn5, Ti40Zr40-Si8-Sn2, Ti40Zr40-Si5-Sn5.

Sample	E_{corr} mV vs AgAgCl	I pass μA.cm^{-2}	E pit mV vs AgAgCl	Epp mV vs AgAgCl	η pit mV
Ti50Zr30-Si8-Sn2	-327.7 ± 16.6	2.84 ± 0.63	993.5 ± 92.2	622.5 ± 33.5	1231.2 ± 108.8
Ti50Zr30-Si5-Sn5	-320.0 ± 40.3	2.37 ± 0.17	674.9 ± 64.2	287.5 ± 35.6	995.0 ±48.1
Ti40Zr40-Si8-Sn2	-333.0 ± 20.0	2.21 ± 0.72	678.5 ± 19.2	350.3 ± 25.1	1010.5 ± 37.8
Ti40Zr40-Si5-Sn5	-335.1 ± 59.4	2.81 ± 0.07	543.3 ± 38.1	255.4 ± 12.6	878.4 ± 77.8

The four ribbons present a passive behavior with similar corrosion potential and passivation current density. But evident differences in some alloys' pitting potential, and repassivation potential are observed.

The similarity of the corrosion potential and passivation current density values indicates that the nature of the passive films formed on the surface of the samples is very comparable, or that the reactivity of these materials in a saline environment is very close (including the passive film formation mechanisms). On the other hand, it is interesting to note that the sensitivity to pitting corrosion as well as the ability to repassivate are different. These results suggest that the chemical composition significantly affects the improvement of the pitting corrosion resistance.

For all the tested materials, the alloys with a higher Ti/Zr ratio tend to have higher pitting and repassivation potentials. Ti alloys are generally protected against corrosion by a passive film mainly composed of Ti-rich oxide, while Zr alloys by a Zr-rich oxide. The increase of the Ti/Zr ratio in the alloy may imply an increase in the Ti content in the passive layer. As Zr oxide is known to be more susceptible to localized breakdown in halide-containing solutions, the overall corrosion resistance of the alloy should be related to the Ti-rich main oxide network [23]. Another trend regards the repartition of soft metals and metalloids. The alloys containing Si and Ge highest content (and consequently Sn and B lowest contents) show an improved passive behavior for the same Ti/Zr ratio. The contribution of these elements to the reactivity or the passive steady state remains under controversy. In the present case, it seems that Si contributes to the stability of the passive state [24]. This assumption will be discussed regarding the passive film chemistry.

Finally, although studied under different conditions, it is important to note that the performance of these alloys is much better than that measured on the previous system.

Immersion Test Results

To confirm the relatively good corrosion resistance of these alloys, immersion tests were performed during four weeks in the saline solution at 37°C. The cumulative ion release (Ti, Zr, Sn, Ge) measured by ICP-MS for the four alloys is represented on Figure 5. It was not possible to quantify Si and B as they are constitutive elements of most of the lab equipment. For Sn and Ge, most of the ion releasing occurs during the first two weeks while for Ti and Zr a continuous releasing is observed. This result suggests that Sn and Ge do not contribute to the passive steady state (steady-state reactions). Titanium is the most released element. The final amount of ions released is almost identical for all materials and remains very low (less than 10 $\mu g.L^{-1}$ even after four weeks of immersion) indicating that these materials have a good corrosion resistance. The ions release is almost negligible when the passive steady state is achieved.

The monitoring of the pH and the mass loss of the samples did not reveal any degradation of the samples. The pH did not change significantly (same for the mass of the samples). After SEM observations of the samples, no evidence of corrosion was detected.

Role of the Alloy Composition on the Passive Film Chemistry and Corrosion Resistance

To better understand the role of the alloy composition, the surface chemistry of the four alloys after 24 h immersed in the 0.9%NaCl solutions was evaluated by XPS. Figure 6 shows a graph of the atomic concentration of the metallic elements detected

Figure 5

Cumulative ions release for Ti50Zr30-Si8-Sn2, Ti50Zr30-Si5-Sn5, Ti40Zr40-Si8-Sn2, Ti40Zr40-Si5-Sn5 over time (from 1 to 4 four weeks of exposure in 0,9%NaCl at 37°C).

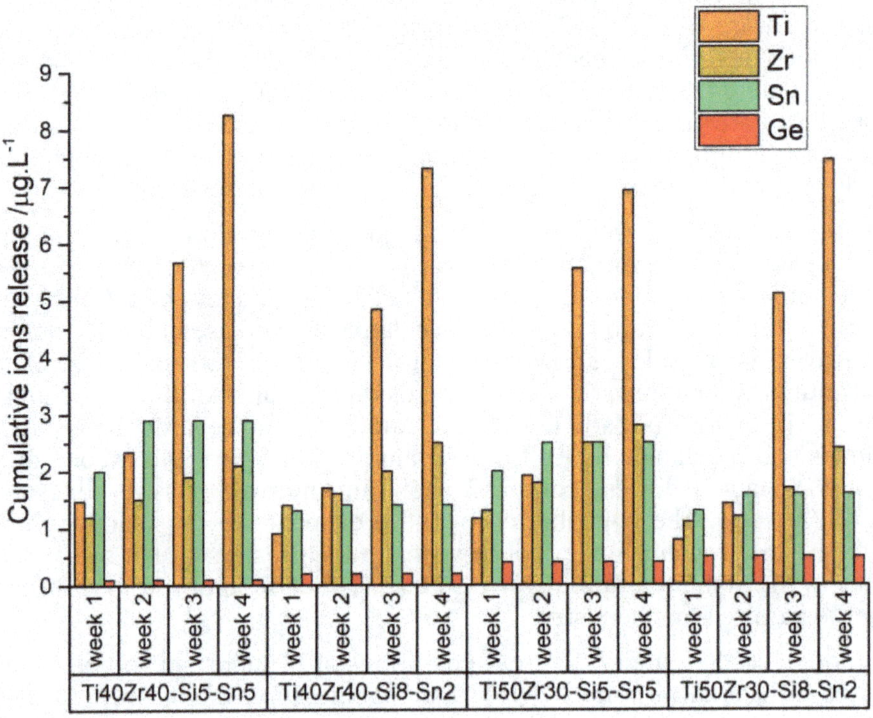

in the passive film for the four alloys. This graph was obtained from the fitting and deconvolution of the high resolution spectrum obtained for Ti (Ti 2p), Zr (Zr 3d), Si (Si 3p), Sn (Sn 3d), respectively. B and Ge were not observed on the passive layer.

Figure 6

Surface metallic oxides concentration (Atomic %) of the samples Ti50Zr30-Si8-Sn2, Ti50Zr30-Si5-Sn5, Ti40Zr40-Si8-Sn2, Ti40Zr40-Si5-Sn5 after 24 h immersed in 0.9 %NaCl at 37°C.

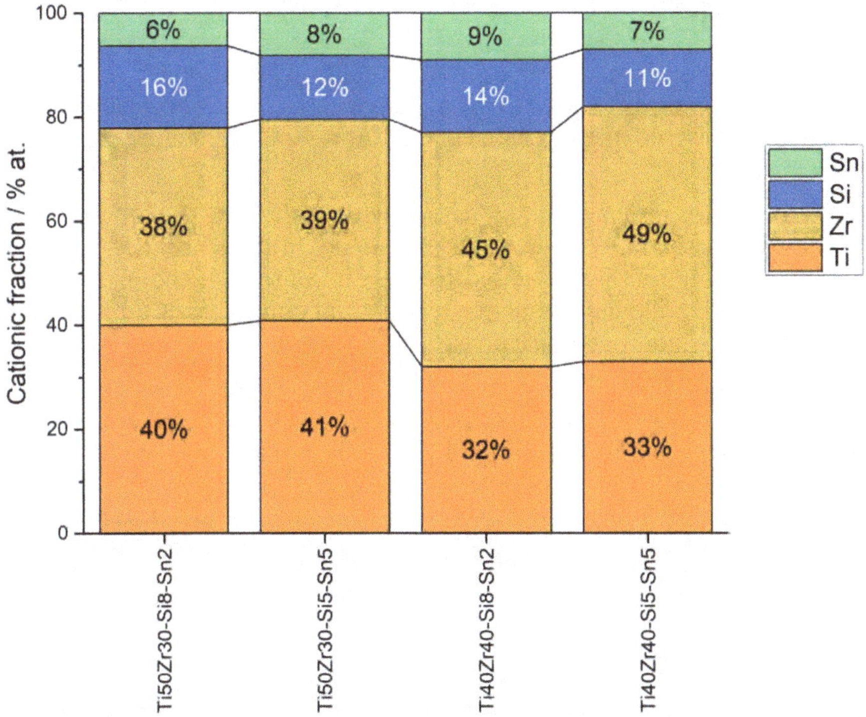

According to the atomic concentration, it can be observed that the passive film is mainly composed of Ti and Zr oxides, followed by Si and Sn oxides. The concentration of Ti in the passive film tends to decrease as the concentration of Zr increases. For all the materials, it was found that the atomic concentration of Zr in the passive layer was higher than in the substrate composition, indicating that Zr is preferentially oxidized. Generally, passive films grown on Ti or Zr alloys in a low-concentration saline solution were stable and less susceptible to pitting corrosion (TA6V polarization curve on Figure 1). This finding suggests that even if the main oxide is Ti and Zr-rich on the tested BMGs, the passive film grown on the BMG is probably more defective than the one of TA6V, for example. The competition between the oxidations of Ti and Zr, as well as the oxidation and dissolution of other alloying elements during the passivation process, may result in the formation of a complex and defective passive film. Furthermore, the chemical modification of the underneath substrate may also limit the repassivation ability of the alloy.

The Si seems to contribute to the passive film chemistry. Sn content is very similar in the different samples' passive films but with a slight tendency to increase in agreement with the Sn content in the alloy. Therefore, Si and Sn play a role in the passive behavior by stabilizing the passive film and reducing the amount of Zr oxide. However, they play a minor role compared with the Ti/Zr ratio in the passive film composition as a function of the Ti/Zr ratio of the substrate[23].

These results suggest that the improved resistance to pitting corrosion is mainly governed by the passive film composition. Increase the Ti/Zr ratio tends to increase the pitting corrosion resistance. However, a compromise needs to be found as an increase of Ti in the alloy composition is detrimental to the GFA.

CONCLUSIONS

This work proposes some guidance to develop metallic glasses applied to the biomedical field. Based on the study of the corrosion behavior of some alloys already studied in the literature and by studying the behavior of four new alloys, some conclusions can be drawn.

Although necessary to obtain metallic glasses with high GFA, the amount of Cu in Ti-based metallic glasses must be minimized. Indeed, in this case, the sensitivity to localized corrosion is directly correlated to the Cu content of the alloy. Moreover, depending on the other alloying elements, it is not uncommon for Cu to promote the precipitation of crystalline secondary phase.

Furthermore, we have seen that the Ti/Zr ratio in the alloy composition plays a major role in the passive behavior of the alloy and in its resistance to pitting corrosion. An optimized Ti and Zr content must be targeted in order to guarantee the glassy state but also a more resistant film to chloride attack. For this purpose, metalloids or soft metals can be added to minimize the Zr content in the passive film or to stabilize it.

The materials studied in this work in ribbon form are being developed in rod to estimate their GFA. First results attesting their biocompatibility have been obtained[18].

ACKNOWLEDGEMENTS

Author thanks A. Liens, L. Gautier, L. Zarazúa-Villalobos, J. Galipaud, J. Chevalier and D. Fabregue from INSA Lyon (Villeurbanne, France) for their technical and scientific support; H. Kato and T. Wada from Tohoku University (Sendai, Japan) for supplying the TiZrCuPd alloys; B. Sarac and E Yuce from Erich Schmid Institute of Materials Science (Leoben, Austria) for supplying the TiZrSiGeBSn alloys. This project was supported by the Agence National de la Research (ANR), Projet-ANR-18-CE91-0005 and for its funding of Labcom 'LEAD' within the framework of ANR-14-LAB5-006, as well as the Austrian Science Fund (FWF) under project grant I3937-N36.

REFERENCES

1. Ali S., Rani A.M.A., Baig Z., Ahmed S.W., Hussain G., Subramaniam K., Hastuty S., Rao T.V.V.L.N., "Biocompatibility and corrosion resistance of metallic biomaterials", *Corros. Rev.* 38 (2020) p. 381.
2. Sarraf M., Rezvani Ghomi E., Alipour S., Ramakrishna S., Liana Sukiman N., "A state-of-the-art review of the fabrication and characteristics of titanium and its alloys for biomedical applications", *Bio-Des. Manuf.* 5 (2022) p. 371.
3. Geetha M., Singh A.K., Asokamani R., Gogia A.K., "Ti based biomaterials, the ultimate choice for orthopaedic implants – A review", *Prog. Mater. Sci.* 54 (2009) p. 397.
4. Li Y., Wong C., Xiong J., Hodgson P., Wen C., "Cytotoxicity of titanium and titanium alloying elements", *J. Dent. Res.* 89 (2010) p. 493.

5. Ridzwan M.I.Z., Shuib S., Hassan A.Y., Shokri A.A. and Mohamad Ibrahim M.N., "Problem of Stress Shielding and Improvement to the Hip Implant Designs: A Review," *Journal of Medical Sciences* 7, 3 (2007) p. 460.
6. Pitchi C.S., Priyadarshini A., Sana G., Narala S.K.R., "A review on alloy composition and synthesis of β-Titanium alloys for biomedical applications", *Mater. Today Proc.* 26 (2020) p. 3297.
7. Hanada S., Ozaki T., Takahashi E., Watanabe S., Yoshimi K., Abumiya T., "Composition Dependence of Young's Modulus in Beta Titanium Binary Alloys," Mater. Sci. Forum. 426–432 (2003) p. 3103.
8. Navarro Laboulais J., Amigó Mata A., Amigó Borrás V., Igual Muñoz A., "Electrochemical characterization and passivation behaviour of new beta-titanium alloys (Ti35Nb10Ta-xFe)", *Electrochimica Acta.* 227 (2017) p. 410.
9. Calin M., Gebert A., Ghinea A.C., Gostin P.F., Abdi S., Mickel C., Eckert J., "Designing biocompatible Ti-based metallic glasses for implant applications", *Mater. Sci. Eng.* C. 33 (2013) p. 875.
10. Zhu S.L., Wang X.M., Qin F.X., Inoue A., "A new Ti-based bulk glassy alloy with potential for biomedical application", *Mater. Sci. Eng.* A. 459 (2007) p. 233.
11. Qin F., Yoshimura M., Wang X., Zhu S., Kawashima A., Asami K., Inoue A., "Corrosion Behavior of a Ti-Based Bulk Metallic Glass and Its Crystalline Alloys", *Mater. Trans.* 48 (2007) p. 1855.
12. Guo Y., Bataev I., Georgarakis K., Jorge A.M., Nogueira R.P., Pons M., Yavari A.R., "Ni- and Cu-free Ti-based metallic glasses with potential biomedical application", *Intermetallics.* 63 (2015) p. 86.
13. Wang Y.B., Li H.F., Cheng Y., Zheng Y.F., Ruan L.Q., "In vitro and in vivo studies on Ti-based bulk metallic glass as potential dental implant material", *Mater. Sci. Eng.* C 33 (2013) p. 3489.
14. Li J., Shi L., Zhu Z., He Q., Ai H., Xu J., "Zr61Ti2Cu25Al12 metallic glass for potential use in dental implants: Biocompatibility assessment by in vitro cellular responses", *Mater. Sci. Eng.* C. 33 (2013) p. 2113.
15. Khan M.M., Nemati A., Rahman Z.U., Shah U.H., Asgar H., Haider W., "Recent Advancements in Bulk Metallic Glasses and Their Applications: A Review", *Crit. Rev. Solid State Mater. Sci.* 43 (2018) p. 233.
16. NF EN ISO 10271:2020, "*Médecine bucco-dentaire – Méthodes d'essai de corrosion des matériaux métalliques*" (AFNOR eds, Fr).
17. Liens A., Ter-Ovanessian B., Courtois N., Fabregue D., Wada T., Kato H., Chevalier J., "Effect of alloying elements on the microstructure and corrosion behavior of TiZr-based bulk metallic glasses", *Corros. Sci.* 177 (2020) #108854.
18. Yüce E., Zarazúa-Villalobos L., Ter-Ovanessian B., Sharifikolouei E., Najmi Z., Spieckermann F., Eckert J., Sarac B., "New-generation biocompatible Ti-based metallic glass ribbons for flexible implants", *Mater. Des.* 223 (2022) #111139.
19. Gautier L., Liens A., Ter-Ovanessian B., Marcelin S., Douillard T., Richard H., Courtois N., Chevalier J., Fabrègue D., "Impact of spherulite-type crystalline defects on the mechanical and electrochemical properties of Ti40Cu36Zr10Pd14 metallic glasses", *Materialia.* 21 (2022) #101353.
20. Gostin P.F., Eigel D., Grell D., Eckert J., Kerscher E., Gebert A., "Comparing the pitting corrosion behavior of prominent Zr-based bulk metallic glasses", *J. Mater. Res.* 30 (2015) p. 233.

21. Wei Q., Gostin P.F., Addison O., Reed D., Calin M., Bera S., Ramasamy P., Davenport A., "The Influence of Partial Replacement of Cu with Ga on the Corrosion Behavior of Ti40Zr10Cu36Pd14 Metallic Glasses", *J. Electrochem. Soc.* 166 (2019) p. C485.
22. Li Y., Xu J., "Role of late transition metals on pitting resistance of Zr-Ti-(Cu, Ni, Co)-Al bulk metallic glasses in 0.6M NaCl aqueous solution", *J. Mater. Sci. Technol.* 33 (2017) p. 1278.
23. Akimoto T., Ueno T., Tsutsumi Y., Doi H., Hanawa T., Wakabayashi N., "Evaluation of corrosion resistance of implant-use Ti-Zr binary alloys with a range of compositions", *J. Biomed. Mater. Res. B Appl. Biomater.* 106 (2018) p. 73.
24. Wang P.-C., Lee J.-W., Yang Y.-C., Lou B.-S., "Effects of silicon contents on the characteristics of Zr–Ti–Si–W thin film metallic glasses", *Thin Solid Films.* 618 (2016) p. 28.

Paper Number:
C2016-07842

Electrochemical Evaluation of Titanium-Boron Alloys for Potential Biomedical Applications

Kristen McCann
California State Polytechnic University

Janice Miguel
California State Polytechnic University

Travis Voorhees
California State Polytechnic University

Vilupanur Ravi
California State Polytechnic University

Gamer Margoosian
California State Polytechnic University

Abstract

Structural biomedical implant alloys are predominantly titanium-based with UNS R56400 (Ti-6Al-4V; Ti64) being the most commonly used. These alloys demonstrate excellent corrosion resistance and biocompatibility; however, there is an ongoing need to have longer lasting implants given the rapid increase in the longevity of the world's population. A critical issue concerning the durability of the implants is aseptic loosening, a phenomenon initiated by the release of metallic cations from the alloy that alters the equilibrium between osteoclasts (bone-consuming cells) and osteoblasts (bone-building cells) and promotes the growth of osteoclasts. One potential approach to alleviating this problem is through the use of alternative alloys that could provide higher durability, e.g., by reducing the release of cations, evoking a more favorable cell response, etc. Recently, titanium alloys containing a moderate amount of boron have been developed for structural applications. In this study, the response of Ti64 with different amounts of boron were characterized in lactated Ringer's solutions, Hank's Balanced Salt Solution and Phosphate Buffered Saline using cyclic potentiodynamic polarization tests based on a modified version of the ASTM F2129-08 test, as well as the ASTM G59-97 testing protocol.

Keywords: corrosion, titanium, boron, structural implant, ASTM F2129-08

INTRODUCTION

Total hip replacement durability is becoming a pressing issue as both the global population and the percentage of the population above the age of 65 are increasing at a rapid rate. According to the United States Centers for Disease Control and Prevention, the number of total hip replacements performed in the United States increased from 138,700 in the year 2000 to 310,800 in the year 2010, more than doubling in ten years.[1] Additionally, the percentage of hip replacement recipients who were under the age 65 at the time of surgery increased from 36% in the year 2000 to 46% in 2010.[1]

The leading type of hip implant failure is known as aseptic loosening[2] which may be caused by an imbalance in cell differentiation and activity of osteoclasts (bone-consuming cells) and osteoblasts (bone-building cells) as a result of an immune-system response to a foreign agent (implant). The equilibrium between osteolysis (resorption of bone by osteoclasts) and ossification (bone formation by osteoblasts) is driven in favor of osteolysis leading to the loosening and subsequent de-bonding of the implant material from its surrounding bone, eventually requiring painful and expensive revision surgery. For older patients, complications can be quite severe.

The leading material used for structural implants is Ti-6Al-4V (Ti64) because of the excellent corrosion resistance, biocompatibility and mechanical properties of this alloy. Titanium forms a passive oxide layer that protects it from the environment. Recent developments have shown that the addition of boron to Ti64 improves mechanical properties such as yield strength and hardness.[3,4,5] The corrosion and biocompatibility studies thus far have been encouraging.[6 - 9] In this paper, further progress on the corrosion study of these alloys is reported in the context of physiologically-relevant media.

EXPERIMENTAL PROCEDURES

Ti64 with boron compositions varying from <0.001 wt% up to 1.09 wt% were cast and hot isostatically pressed (C+HIP). Test coupons were cut out from the alloy billets using electrical discharge machining (EDM). The coupons were ground using 240, 320, 400, 600, and 800 silicon carbide grit paper and then polished with oil and diamond paste with particle sizes of 6, 3, and 1 μm. The final surface finish was obtained using 0.05 μm alumina polish in water. Finally, the test coupons were ultrasonically cleaned using deionized water, alcohol, and again deionized water for three minutes each.

Test coupons were subjected to a modified ASTM F2129-08 "Standard Test Method for Conducting Cyclic Potentiodynamic Polarization Measurements to Determine the Corrosion Susceptibility of Small Implant Devices" standard test. Sibling coupons were characterized using ASTM G59-97 "Standard Test Method for Conducting Potentiodynamic Polarization Resistance Measurements" standard. These tests were conducted in a three-electrode flat cell using a Ag/AgCl reference electrode with 3M NaCl filling solution (+209 mV vs. SHE) and a platinum-coated niobium mesh counter electrode. The working electrode, i.e., the test coupon, had an exposed surface area of 1 cm^2. Tests were carried out in three different physiological solutions: phosphate buffered saline (PBS) [nominally 0.800 g/L NaCl, 0.020 g/L KCl, 0.115 g/L Na_2HPO_4, and 0.020 g/L KH_2PO_4], Hank's balanced salt solution (Hank's) [nominally 0.7998 g/L NaCl, 0.0400 g KCl, 0.0090 g/L $NaH_2PO_4 \cdot 7H_2O$, 0.0186 g/L $CaCl_2 \cdot 2H_2O$, 0.0200 g/L $MgSO_4 \cdot 7H_2O$, 0.035 g/L $NaHCO_3$, 0.0060 g/L KH_2PO_4, 0.1000 g/L glucose], and lactated Ringer's solution (Ringer's) [nominally 0.860 g/L NaCl, 0.033 g/L $CaCl_2$, and 0.030 g/L KCl], 10% donor bovine blood serum [nominally 25 mL donor bovine serum mixed with 225 mL 0.9 wt% NaCl solution to make 250 mL of overall solution]. Each of these solutions were made with 18•MΩ-cm double deionized water.

Cyclic Potentiodynamic Polarization (CPP) Scans

One of the test protocols followed was a modified ASTM F2129-08 standard testing method. The two modifications to this test were (1) the use of 250 mL solution instead of 500 mL and (2) a Ag/AgCl [3M NaCl] reference electrode instead of a saturated calomel electrode (SCE). The solution was heated to 37°C and deaerated with nitrogen for 30 minutes prior to the start of the test. The temperature was maintained throughout the test with a heating jacket and deaeration was continued. Open circuit potentials (OCP) were recorded for one hour followed by cyclic potentiodynamic polarization. The applied potential was raised from the OCP to an apex value of 800 mV (vs. Ag/AgCl [3M NaCl]) at a scanning rate of 0.167 mV/s and then reversed back down to the OCP value at the same rate.

Upon completion of the modified ASTM F2129-08 test, the potential and current density values at the intersection of the tangents to the anodic and cathodic portions were determined. Due to the nature of the test, these were post-passivation values. It should be noted that since the ASTM F2129-08 testing standard calls for a SCE electrode (+241 mV vs. SHE), and a Ag/AgCl [3M NaCl] electrode (+209 mV vs. SHE) was used for the tests in this paper, the potential readings can be converted by subtracting 32 mV from the value of interest.

Corrosion rate is directly proportional to the corrosion current density, and can be determined using the following equation:

$$CR = 3.27 \times 10^{-3} \frac{EW i_{corr}}{\rho}$$

Where, CR is the corrosion rate in mm/year, EW is the equivalent weight of the corroding coupon in grams, i_{corr} is the corrosion current density (nA/cm^2), and ρ is the density of the corroding material in g/cm^3.

Linear Polarization Resistance Scans

A linear polarization resistance (LPR) scan was run upon the completion of one hour of OCP for a polished and ground coupon. This scan applied a small perturbation voltage from -40 mV to +40 mV vs. OCP and measured the responding current. The same scan rate, cell geometry, solution temperature, volume, exposed surface area and reference electrode were kept constant as per the modified ASTM F2129-08 test. The three solutions used with this test were phosphate buffered saline (created using the procedure previously stated), normal saline (0.9 wt% NaCl solution), and 10% donor bovine blood serum (25 mL donor bovine serum mixed with 225 mL 0.9 wt% NaCl solution to make 250 mL of overall solution).

The results from this test were plotted as voltage (with reference to Ag/AgCl [3M NaCl]) vs. current density which results in a linear sloped line. By taking the slope of the line at zero current, the resistance polarization can be found based on Ohm's law: V = IR, rearranged to form: $R = \frac{V}{I}$. This value describes the resistance of the alloy to entering into a state of oxidation or reduction. This value is similar to a charge transfer resistance and is inversely proportional to corrosion rate.

Potentiodynamic Polarization Tests

Immediately following the linear polarization resistance scan, a potentiodynamic polarization (Tafel test) scan was applied from -400 to +400 mV vs. OCP. The corrosion potentials and corrosion current densities were obtained from the Tafel region. It is to be noted that these data are representative of the alloy prior to passivation – a reasonable assumption given the short duration of the exposure (8 minutes) and small perturbation voltages.

RESULTS

In this section, the results from the different test protocols described above will be described. The results are divided into separate sections for ease of readability.

Figure 1a

Modified F2129-08 tests run in lactated Ringer's solution for Ti64 with varying amounts of boron (up to 0.04 wt% B).

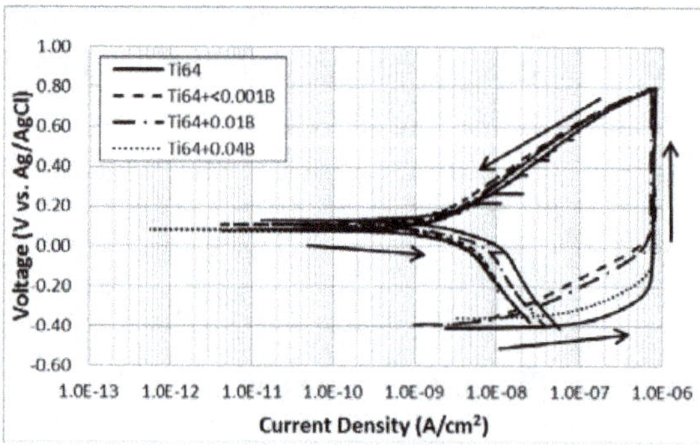

Figure 1b

Modified F2129-08 tests run in lactated Ringer's solution for Ti64 with varying amounts of boron (> 0.04 wt% B).

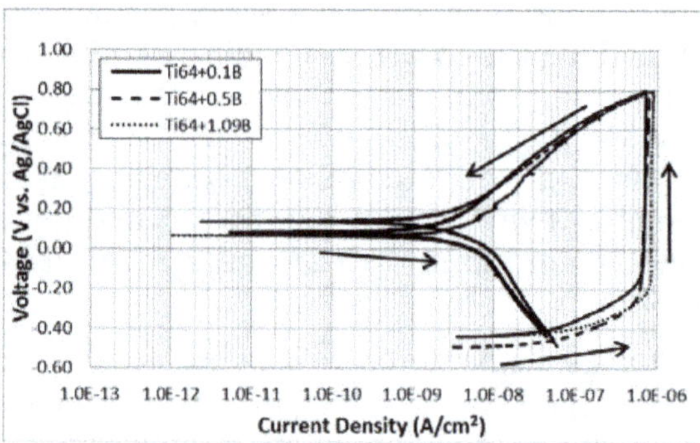

Modified F2129-08

Lactated Ringer's Solution

Cyclic potentiodynamic polarization scans were run according to the modified ASTM F2129-08 in lactated Ringer's solution (Figures 1a and 1b). The results show that all of the alloys tested passed the test with no evidence of pitting. There were differences in the onset of passivation, i.e., the passivation potentials, with no clear trend in regards to boron additions. The results (Table 1) show that the post-passivation corrosion potential of the alloys in lactated Ringer's solution drops (in general) with increasing boron contents with a notable exception at the 0.5 wt% B level. The corrosion current density values seem to decrease initially for ultralow boron levels before increasing again; however, these values were extremely low overall (2 – 4 nA/cm^2) with the exception of the 1 wt% B alloy. This is further illustrated by the corrosion rate calculations, the results of which are displayed in the last column. At the apex of the graphs in Figures 1a and 1b the current densities shift to the left, indicating that no pitting occurred. This was confirmed by optical microscopy. Since none of the alloys pitted in this test, they are all considered potential candidates for biomedical applications according to this standard.

Figure 2a

Modified F2129-08 tests run in Hank's solution for Ti64 with varying amounts of boron.

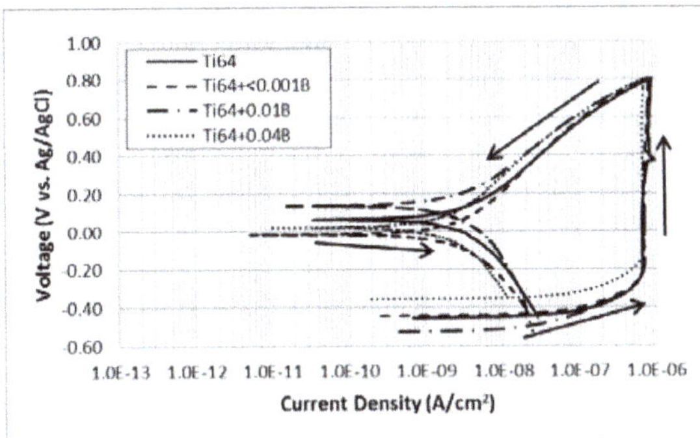

Figure 2b

Modified F2129-08 tests run in Hank's solution for Ti64 with varying amounts of boron.

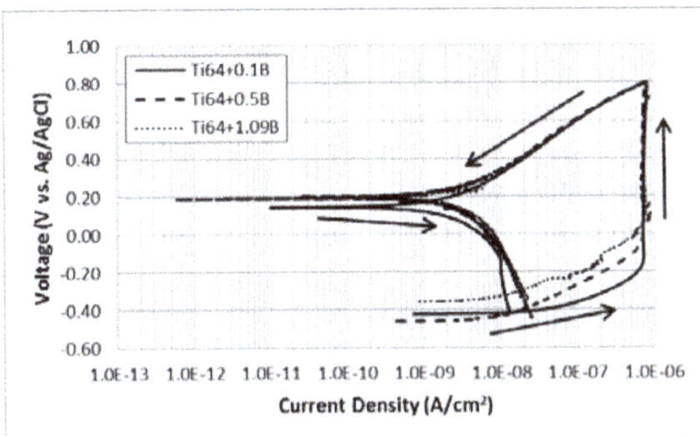

Table 1

Post passivation corrosion behavior of alloys from modified F2129-08 in lactated Ringer's solution.

Alloy	Corrosion Potential (mV vs. E_{ref})	Corrosion Current Density (nA/cm^2)	Corrosion Rate (μm/year)
Ti64	129.0	3.800	67.2
Ti64 + < 0.001B	109.0	1.907	33.7
Ti64 + 0.01B	104.0	2.430	41.1
Ti64 + 0.04B	84.2	3.090	52.3
Ti64 + 0.1B	84.9	3.317	56.1
Ti64 + 0.5B	138.7	3.840	64.9
Ti64 + 1.09B	66.3	12.51	210.9

Figure 3a

Modified F2129-08 tests run in phosphate buffered saline for Ti64 with varying amounts of boron.

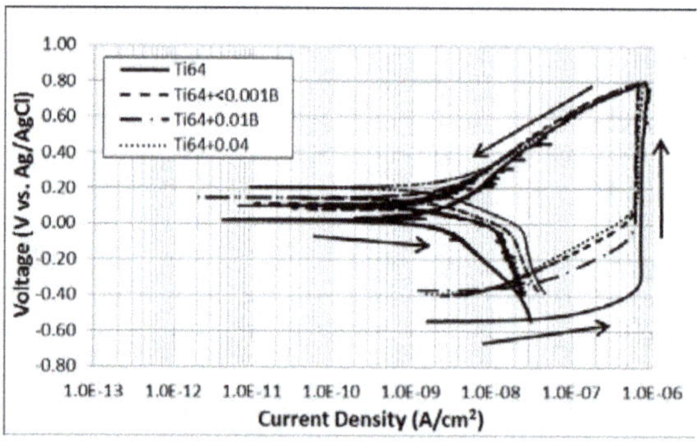

Hank's Solution

Cyclic potentiodynamic polarization scans were run according to modified ASTM F2129-08 in Hank's solution as well (Figures 2a and 2b). No pitting was observed in any alloys as well under these test conditions indicating all alloy compositions passed this test. The results (Table 2) showed a general increase in post-passivation corrosion potential, i.e., increased nobility, as the boron content increased with two notable exceptions (< 0.001 and 0.04 wt% B). The corrosion potential values ranged from -20.1 to 194.5 mV vs. Ag/AgCl [3M NaCl]. The corrosion current density values generally decreased for all B containing alloys relative to the base alloy with the notable exception of the 0.04 wt% B alloy. This is more clearly seen in the corrosion rate column, with a significant drop for the 0.01 wt% B alloy. However, in general, all of the corrosion rates are low.

Phosphate Buffered Saline

Cyclic potentiodynamic polarization scans were also run according to modified ASTM F2129-08 in Phosphate Buffered Saline (Figures 3a and 3b). Again, none of the alloys showed pitting behavior. There is a general increase in the nobility of the alloys as

Table 2

Post Passivation corrosion behavior of alloys from modified F2129-08 in Hank's Solution.

Alloy	Corrosion Potential (mV vs. E_{ref})	Corrosion Current Density (nA/cm^2)	Corrosion Rate (μm/year)
Ti64	64.0	5.590	98.8
Ti64 + < 0.001B	-15.4	4.483	79.3
Ti64 + 0.01B	135.0	4.020	8.0
Ti64 + 0.04B	-20.1	8.630	146.0
Ti64 + 0.1B	144.0	3.710	62.8
Ti64 + 0.5B	193.0	4.090	69.1
Ti64 + 1.09B	194.5	3.350	56.5

Figure 3b

Modified F2129-08 tests run in phosphate buffered saline for Ti64 with varying amounts of boron.

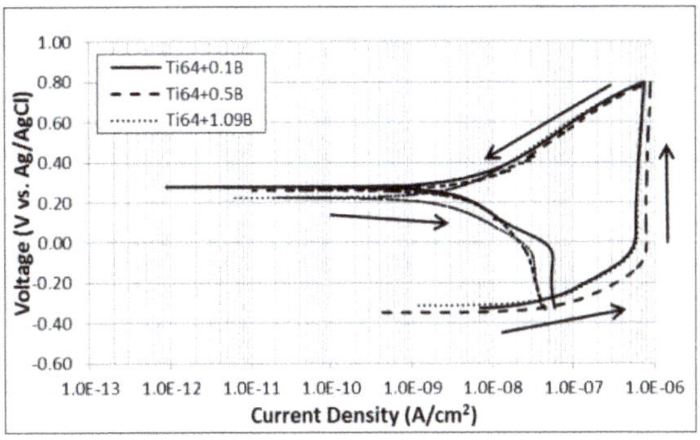

the boron content is increased. The corrosion current densities (Table 3) and the corresponding corrosion rates show an initial decrease as the boron content increases to 0.04 wt% B. At the higher B contents, the increases are more pronounced (0.1 and 0.5 wt% B) followed by a decrease at 1 wt% B.

Linear Polarization Resistance (LPR)

Phosphate Buffered Saline

The polarization resistance of the alloy can be determined with the LPR test using Ohm's law, (V=IR). Figures 4a and 4b show the potential Vs current density plots for Ti64 alloys with different B contents. Table 4 presents the polarization resistance as a function of the B content in PBS. All of the B-containing alloys have a higher polarization resistance in comparison to the base alloy with the values ranging from 420 – 1134 kΩ . Similar trends were observed in saline solutions.

Table 3

Post passivation corrosion behavior of alloys from modified F2129-08 in Phosphate Buffered Saline.

Alloy	Corrosion Potential (mV vs. E_{ref})	Corrosion Current Density (nA/cm^2)	Corrosion Rate (μm/ year)
Ti64	22.8	3.617	63.9
Ti64 + < 0.001B	104.0	2.020	35.7
Ti64 + 0.01B	147.7	2.843	48.1
Ti64 + 0.04B	204.0	3.423	57.9
Ti64 + 0.1B	277.7	7.303	123.6
Ti64 + 0.5B	262.0	5.987	101.1
Ti64 + 1.09B	223.0	3.890	65.6

Figure 4a

LPR run in PBS for Ti64 with varying amounts of boron.

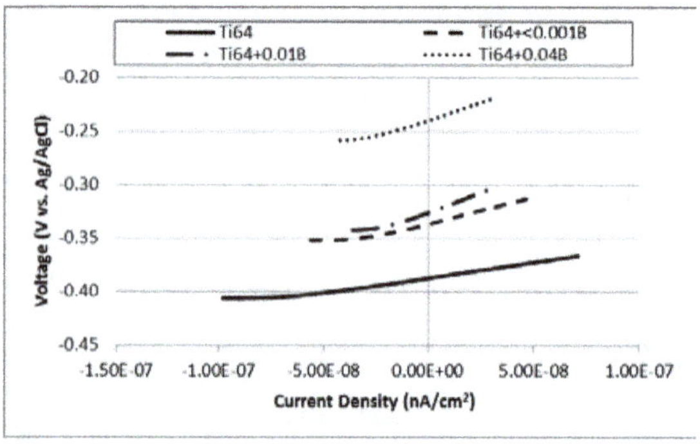

Figure 4b

LPR run in PBS for Ti64 with varying amounts of boron.

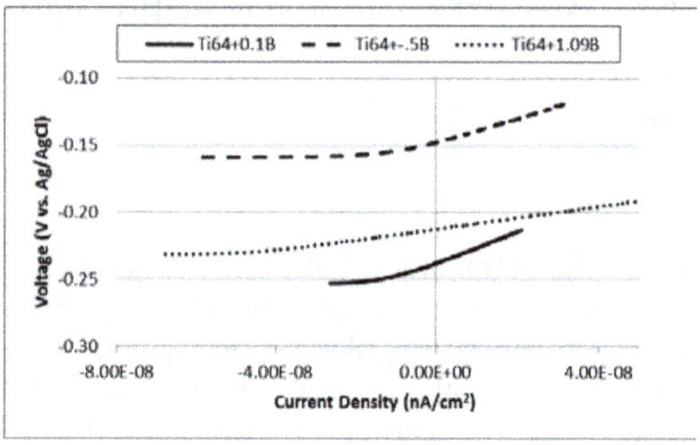

Bovine Blood Serum

Figures 5a and 5b show the potential Vs current density plots for Ti64 alloys containing different amounts of boron in 10% donor bovine blood serum. Table 5 shows that the polarization resistance values increase from Ti64 base alloy to Ti64 + <0.001B, but then decrease as the boron content is increased further, with the exception of Ti64 + 0.5B.

Table 4

Polarization resistance values from LPR run in PBS.

Alloy	Polarization Resistance (kΩ)
Ti64	287.7
Ti64 + < 0.001B	495.9
Ti64 + 0.01B	718.5
Ti64 + 0.04B	637.5
Ti64 + 0.1B	1134
Ti64 + 0.5B	867.4
Ti64 + 1.09B	420.1

Figure 5a

LPR run in 10% donor bovine blood serum for titanium with varying amounts of boron.

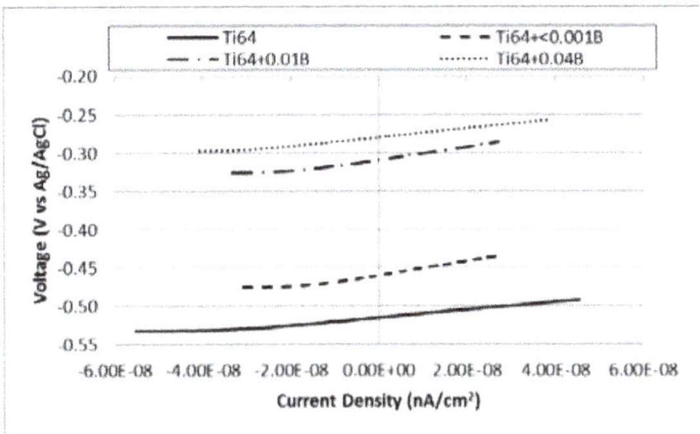

Figure 5b

LPR run in 10% donor bovine blood serum for titanium with varying amounts of boron.

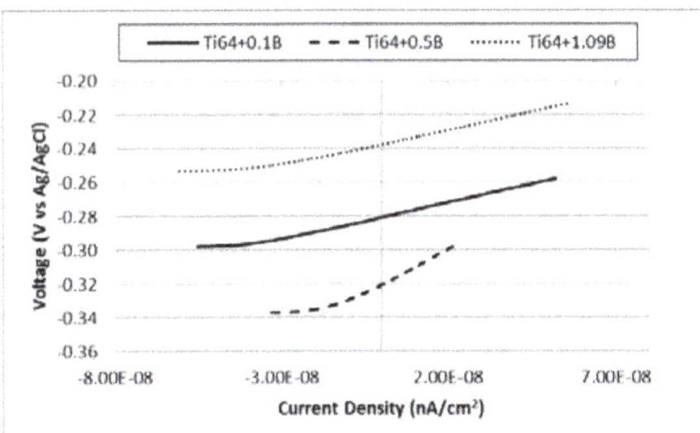

Potentiodynamic Polarization Tests

Potentiodynamic polarization scans were run to further determine corrosion behavior in phosphate buffered saline. This test was run to determine the corrosion potentials and corrosion current densities prior to passivation of the alloys. The results showed

Table 5

Polarization resistance values from LPR run in 10% donor bovine blood serum.

Alloy	Polarization Resistance (kΩ)
Ti64	515.0
Ti64 + < 0.001B	925.3
Ti64 + 0.01B	840.5
Ti64 + 0.04B	581.6
Ti64 + 0.1B	436.6
Ti64 + 0.5B	1010
Ti64 + 1.09B	431.6

Figure 6a

Tafel test run in PBS for titanium with varying amount of boron.

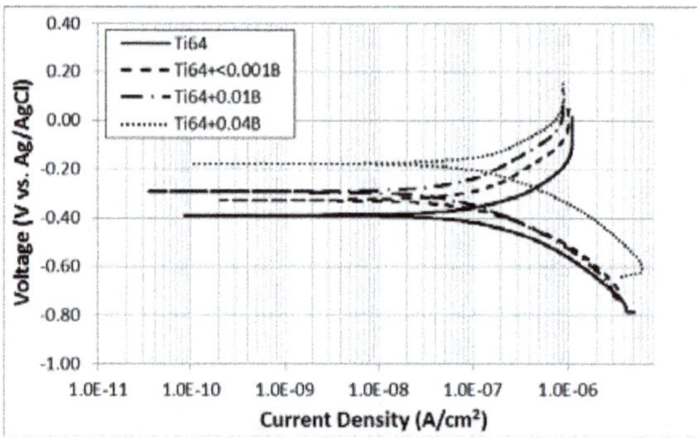

Figure 6b

Tafel test run in PBS for titanium with varying amounts of boron.

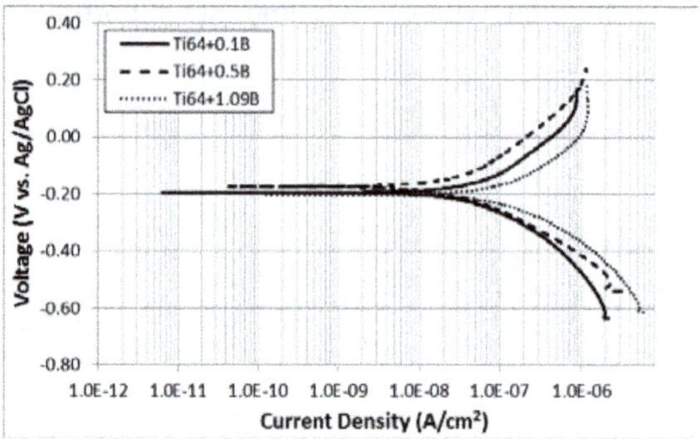

that all B-containing alloys have a higher corrosion potential relative to the base alloy. The corrosion current densities generally decreased as the boron content increased with the notable exception of the 0.1 wt% B alloy.

Table 6

Corrosion behavior of alloys from Tafel test in phosphate buffered saline.

Corrosion Potential (mV vs. E_{ref})	Alloy	Corrosion Current Density (nA/cm^2)	Corrosion Rate (μm/year)
-388	Ti64	1.990	20.1
-301	Ti64 + < 0.001B	1.433	24.6
-327	Ti64 + 0.01B	1.467	24.8
-292	Ti64 + 0.04B	0.943	16.0
-177	Ti64 + 0.1B	2.073	35.1
-196	Ti64 + 0.5B	0.592	10.1
-176	Ti64 + 1.09B	0.281	4.7

CONCLUSIONS

Cyclic potentiodynamic polarization tests were conducted for titanium and titanium alloys in PBS, Hank's and Ringer's solutions using a modified version of ASTM F2129-08. Linear polarization resistance and potentiodynamic polarization test were performed to further investigate the corrosion behavior of these alloys prior to passivation.

All of the B-containing alloys passed the modified F2129-08 tests in PBS and lactated Ringer's and Hank's solutions. None of these alloys showed any evidence of pitting. Those run in PBS show a general increase in corrosion potential (post-passivation) as the boron content in the alloy was increased up to 0.1 wt% B and thereafter showed a decrease for the 0.5 and 1 wt% B alloys. The tests in Ringer's and PBS show an initial decrease in corrosion current densities with increasing boron content up to 0.01 wt%. The corrosion current density increased as the boron content was further increased. However, all of the current densities recorded were quite low and with few exceptions were in the 2 – 4 nA/cm^2 range and consequently the corrosion rates are quite low.

The linear polarization scans conducted in PBS showed that the addition of <0.001 and 0.01 wt% boron resulted in an increase in the calculated polarization resistance, Rp, of the alloy, relative to its base alloy Ti64, in all solutions tested. The addition of 0.01 wt% boron appears to increase the polarization resistance of the alloy relative to the <0.001 wt% boron base alloy in PBS. The Rp values calculated from tests conducted in PBS continued to increase in magnitude for the 0.01 and 0.04 wt% boron levels. This suggests that the polarization resistance of titanium alloys increases with increasing boron content up to the point where TiB precipitates begin to form in the titanium matrix (estimated to be in the 0.02 – 0.03 wt% range). It is to be noted that all of the polarization resistance values are high (>105 kΩ), further showing that all of the alloys exhibit excellent corrosion resistance.

The pre-passivation potentiodynamic polarization scans show a general increase in corrosion potential when tested in PBS. This shows that the addition of ultra-low concentrations of boron to titanium alloys increases the nobility of the parent alloy. In addition, the corrosion potentials for 10% bovine blood serum and PBS were observed to be higher than those for 0.9 wt% NaCl (data not reported here) pointing to the fact that adding buffers and proteins to saline results in an increase in the measured corrosion potentials of titanium and its alloys.

The corrosion current densities calculated using the potentiodynamic polarization tests in PBS show that the addition of 0.01 wt% boron results in a lower corrosion rate in comparison to the base alloy (<0.001 wt% B) boron and additions of boron ≥0.04 wt%. This suggests that the addition of boron within the solubility range of boron in Ti64 (estimated to be in the 0.02 – 0.03 wt% range) improves both the nobility and corrosion rate of the parent Ti64 alloy.

The above conclusions should be treated as preliminary because of the limited set of samples that were tested. Extensive testing is underway to develop a strong statistical basis for the performance of these alloys in different solutions.

ACKNOWLEDGEMENTS

We would also like to thank Shay McCarthy, Nina Rastogi, Kevin Robles, Obed Villalpando, Mr. Ulus Ekerman & David La Fey (Cal Poly Pomona). We gratefully acknowledge financial support from the LA section of NACE International, Western

States Corrosion Seminar, Western Area of NACE International, NACE Foundation, California Steel Industries, the Southern California Chapter of AIST, Dan Cook & Joyce Barnhurst (Gamry Instruments).

REFERENCES

1. "*Inpatient Surgeries.*" Centers for Disease Control and Prevention. Centers for Disease Control and Prevention, (2014).
2. Donachie M.. *Titanium: A Technical Guide*, 2nd Edition. Materials Park: ASM International, (2000): p. 1.
3. Tsang H.T., Chao C. G., Ma C. Y., "Effects of volume fraction of reinforcement on tensile and creep properties of in-situ TiB/Ti MMC," *Scripta Materialia* 37(9) (1997): p. 1359-1365.
4. Sen I., Tamirisakandala S., Miracle D.B., Ramamurty U., "Microstructural effects on the mechanical behavior of B- modified Ti-6Al-4V alloys," *Acta Materialia* 55 (15) (2007): p. 4983.
5. Ravi V., Schissler A., Chantrjaroen W., Beecher C., Razzak A., Urak R., Alas S., "Corrosion Behaviour and Biocompatibility of Boron Containing Titanium Alloys in Simulated Physiological Environments," *Corrosion Engineering, Science and Technology* 47(5)(2012): p. 383.
6. Ravi V., et al., "Corrosion and Immune Response Of Boron-Modified Titanium Alloys In Biological Environments," Corrosion 2009 Conference & Expo, NACE International. Paper No. 09466 (2009): p. 1.

   Ravi V., Rogers S., Malek M., Surmenian D., Priddy I., Harrison B., Schissler A., Divi Suresh C., Tamirisakandala Sesh, and Miracle Daniel "The environmental stability of boron-containing titanium alloys for biomedical applications," JOM, 63 (6) (2011): p. 42.
7. Voorhees T., Villalpando O. and Ravi V., "Characterization of the Corrosion Behavior of Advanced Titanium Alloys in Simulated Physiological Environments Using Electrochemical Impedance Spectroscopy," Corrosion/2015, NACE, Dallas, TX, Paper No. 6120 (C2015-6120) (2015).
8. Ravi V., Castaneda S., Rey G., Permana B, Wantah W., Morin K., Alas S., Tamirisa S., and Miracle D., "Corrosion and Immune Response Of Advanced Titanium Alloys In Biological Environments," CORROSION/2009, NACE, Atlanta, Paper No. 7500 (2012).
9. Ravi V., Enriquez R. Jr., Beecher C. , Razzak A. , Chantrjaroen W. , Schissler A. , Malek M. , Surmenian D., Priddy I., Urak R., Schooley A. and Alas S., "Stability of advanced titanium alloys in saline solution and characterization of osteoblast activation", Corrosion/2012, NACE, Salt Lake City, Paper No. C2012-0001709 (2012).

Paper Number:
C2017-09271

Bio-Functional High Performance Coatings of Titanium and Magnesium Alloys for Biomedical Applications

Amir Eliezer
Corrosion Research Center

Cyrille Gasqueres
aap Implantate AG

Abstract

Over the past few years, progress in orthopedic surgery has helped to improve the quality of life. Approximately 4.5 million procedures related to joint replacement and fracture repair are performed worldwide each year. However, serious complications still occur mostly due to implant loosening or infection. Surface treatments and coatings have been major research axes to address those problems. In this study, bio-active oxide coating containing silver particles on a titanium medical grade Ti-6Al-4V alloy and the development of a CaP bio-active oxide coating are reported. Both materials coatings were obtained by Plasma Electrolytic Oxidation (PEO). Corrosion of magnesium W4 alloy was investigated in vitro by electrochemical methods in solutions replicating the body's environment. In addition also gas formation of W4 was also quantified. In order to correlate in-vitro corrosion to in-vivo degradation animal studies were performed. A dedicated approach to identify and construct suitable traumatological implants made of magnesium was also undertaken and a suitable manufacturing process on an industrial scale was established. The results lead to the conclusion that in order to effectively tailor and control the biodegradation of titanium and magnesium implants, bio active PEO coatings are essential for biomedical implants.

Keywords: Magnesium, Titanium, PEO, Coatings, innovation, in vitro, in vivo

INTRODUCTION

The major question of the study refers to the fact that up to date it is very difficult to find or define the correlation of corrosion behavior between the human body-scale to the laboratory scale. Another concern is should we consider the human body as an electrochemical cell or we can rely on an electrochemical software for developing biomedical applications.

The lecture will focus on the in-vitro-in-vivo and will present the importance of applied corrosion methods for biomaterials applications. The study will present a dedicated approach to identify and construct suitable traumatological implants made of magnesium as well as was undertaken and a suitable manufacturing process on an industrial scale was established. The results lead to the conclusion that in order to effectively tailor and control the biodegradation of titanium and magnesium implants, for example smart coatings and high tech corrosion approach are valuable to achieve innovative biomedical-devices.

EXPERIMENTAL PROCEDURE

Ti-6Al-4V alloy rods (4.5 mm diameter × 30 mm length) and disks (13 mm diameter × 4 mm height) were cut from medical grade Ti-6Al-4V bar. Cannulated Interference W4 (96% magnesium, 4% yttrium) screws and their runners which were produced by die casting were investigated under in-vitro (electrochemical and gas formation experiments) and in-vivo (sheep) conditions.

The electrochemical measurements were under 0.9% NaCl solution and corrosion was quantified electrochemically by electrochemical impedance spectroscopy (EIS).

The experimental setup for EIS consisted of a unique bio-reactor system in which the key parameters of the milieu were adjusted together with a separate electrochemical cell, in which measurements were made. In order to mimic the tissue conditions as closely as possible the coating solution was adjusted to 36.5–40 C° and pH 7.35–7.45. The flow rate of the solution between the reactor (3000 ml) and the electrochemical cell (500 ml) was chosen to be -100 ml/min and the stirring rate inside the electrochemical cell was 300 ml/min. The parameters were measured using three standard electrodes in an electrochemical cell with a calomel reference electrode and a Pt counter electrode.

The coating topography was investigated by scanning electron microscopy (SEM) using a Philips XL30 ESEM-FEG equipped with a Genisis energy-dispersive X-ray spectrometer (EDS) from EDAX. A PHI 5500 XPS spectrometer with a monochromatic Al Kα radiation was used to analyze the chemical composition of the coating. Chemical binding in the topmost nm of the sample surface was also recorded. Depth profiling was performed using a 3 keV Ar ion beam for sputtering.

To investigate the antibacterial efficacy of the coating, samples were challenged with the gram positive *Staphylococcus epidermidis* strain (ATCC 35984). The microorganisms were cultured in Caso-Bouillon broth at 37°C for 12-16 h (overnight culture) and diluted to 10^6 CFU/ml. 1 ml of the inoculum was incubated with coated and uncoated rods for 3 h, 12 h and 18 h at 37°C under static conditions. Additional HA Coatings were applied on the magnesium alloys using PEO coatings. Both HA and Silver coating required an innovative approach once the leading point was understanding the need of such coatings to extend the lifetime performance in regards to the material and coating biomedical bio active performance.

RESULTS

The Ti-6Al-4V alloy has showed a bio-active anti-bacteria behavior for the coating containing silver particles. The silver coating is intended to prevent colonization of the implant, which is the first step in biofilm formation and in turn for biofilm-related infections. This is a benefit in patients in whom implant-related infections occur particularly frequently as e.g. in open fractures, revision surgery or in patients with an impaired immune system. The coating is not thought to replace but rather to complement antibiotics as the latter are mostly ineffective against biofilms and are of limited use in biofilm prevention.

The SEM images in chemical contrast mode show the presence of a heavy element on the coating surface (bright areas on Figure 1b). Energy-dispersive spectrometry confirms that this heavy element is indeed silver (data not shown). SEM images recorded on various locations of the implant reveal that silver is spread almost homogeneously over the entire coating surface. The size of a typical silver-containing area is below 200 nm (Figure 1a).

The number of adherent *S. epidermidis* bacteria on Ti-alloy, Ag and coated rods were quantified by direct plating (Figure. 2). After 3 h of incubation the Ti-alloy rods already show an extensive colonization of their surfaces. Bacterial numbers (colony-forming unit) were found significantly lower on the pure Ag-rods. The lowest numbers of bacteria were found on the coated surfaces. After 12 h of incubation a lower amount of

Figure 1

High resolution SEM micrographs of the coating in (a) topography contrast mode and (b) chemical contrast mode.

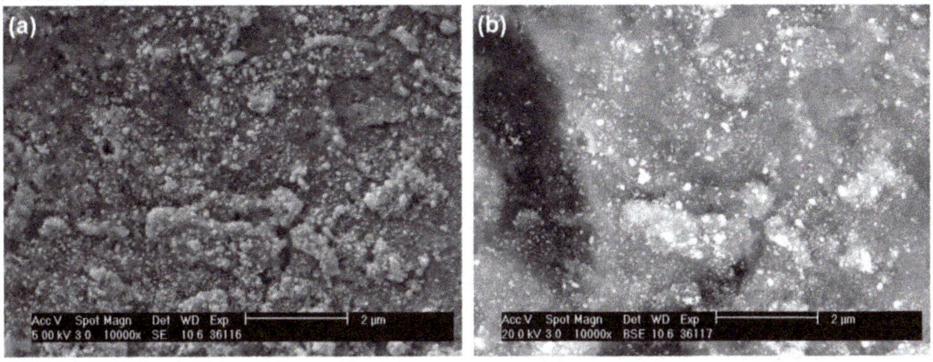

Figure 2

Number of adherent bacteria found on the surface of coated and uncoated Titanium alloy rods and pure silver rods after incubation for 3 h, 12 h and 18 h.

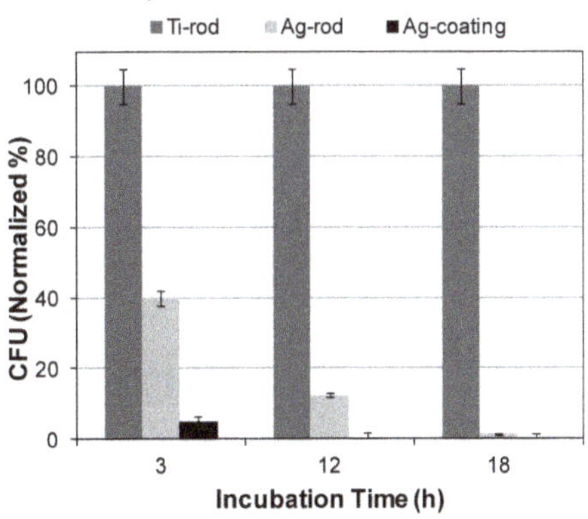

adherent bacteria were found on the pure silver surfaces, meanwhile no living adherent bacteria were found on the coated surfaces, revealing a complete killing of the adherent bacteria. Interestingly, no surviving bacteria were found in the liquid medium in which the coated rods were incubated. The silver ions released from the coating surface have even killed all the planktonic bacteria present in the culture medium. After 18 h of incubation, no surviving bacteria were found on either the pure silver surfaces or the coated surfaces.

The in-vitro measurements showed a significant decrease in corrosion for the W4 PEO coated samples compared to the uncoated samples by up to 90% both in EIS and gas formation. It was shown that PEO coating of W4 screws resulted in a relative improvement of gas formation in-vivo both after 6 and 12 weeks of implantation. Figures 3a to 4b show the results of a physico-chemical characterization (according to ISO/TS 10993-19:2006). In these figures the colloid-dispersed apatite is identified as HA. In detail, Figures 3a-b show an SEM image of the HA coating in chemical contrast mode without or only a low amount of nano-HA (3a) and an EDX spectrum of the bright region indicated by the tip of the arrow (3b). Figures 4a-b show corresponding figures for the HA coating according to the invention. The presence of HA in the

Figure 3

SEM image of the HA basic coating in chemical contrast mode (a), an EDX spectra of the bright region indicated by the tip of the arrow (b).

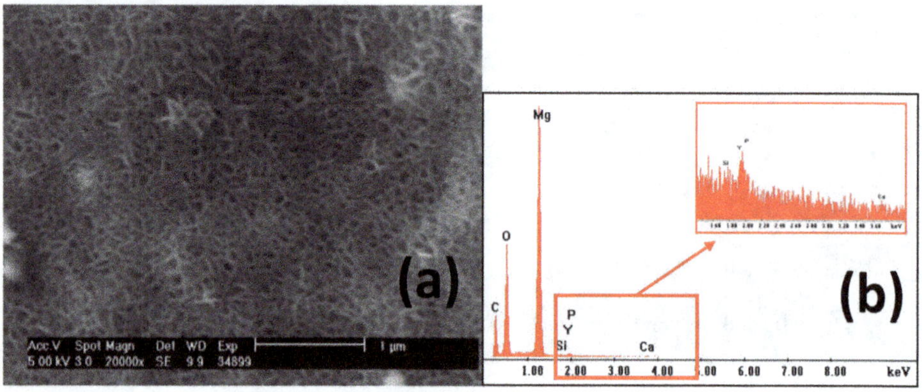

Figure 4

SEM image of the HA upgraded coating in chemical contrast mode (a), an EDX spectra of the bright region indicated by the tip of the arrow (b).

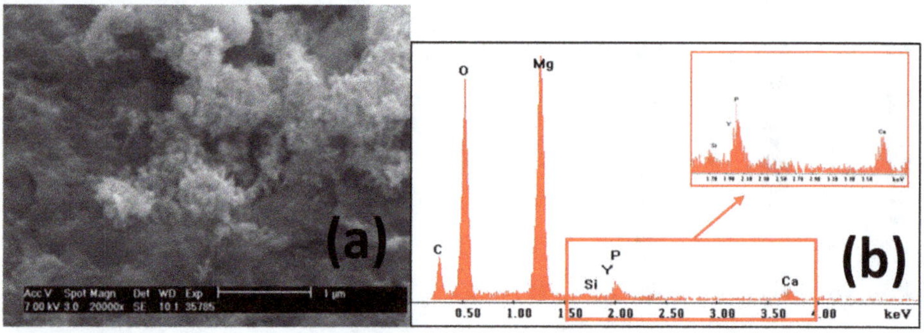

dispersed system seems to be necessary for the formation of HA on the converted surface. The purpose of an apatite-coating is the adaptation and/or the retardation of degradation, in particular the initial degradation. The initial degradation represents the occurring bio-degradation of a bio-degradable implant immediately or directly after implantation.

The in-vitro measurements showed a significant decrease in corrosion for the W4 PEO coated samples compared to the uncoated samples by up to 90% both in EIS and gas formation. It was also shown that PEO coating of W4 screws resulted in a relative improvement of gas formation in-vivo both after 6 and 12 weeks after implantation. The initial degradation represents the occurring bio-degradation of a biodegradable implant immediately or directly after implantation. Figure 5 shows a relative surface biomedical protected controlled layer as experienced under 0-24 hours of electrochemical exposures. Figure 6 shows the smooth HA coated bar.

Figure 5

Electrochemical Impedance Spectroscopy of coated bar-samples, measured into 0.9% NaCl solution (with NaOH, with circulation of electrolyte FR=100 ml/min). Experiment conditions: T=36-37°C; pH=7.4-7.8.

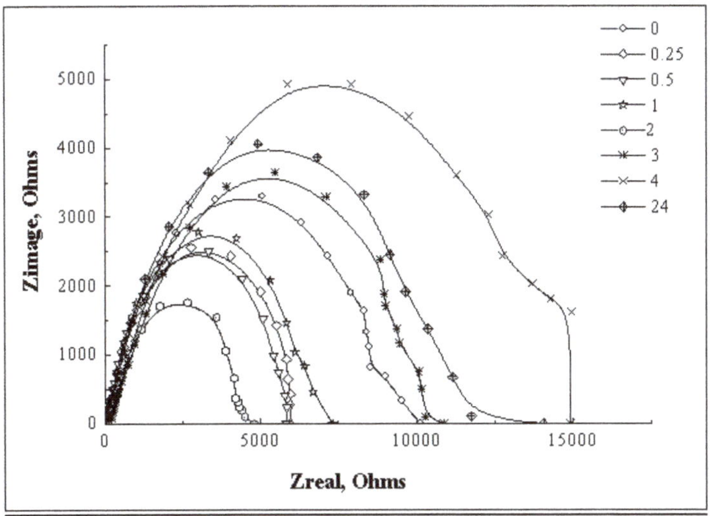

Figure 6

Example of the HA W4 coated bar.

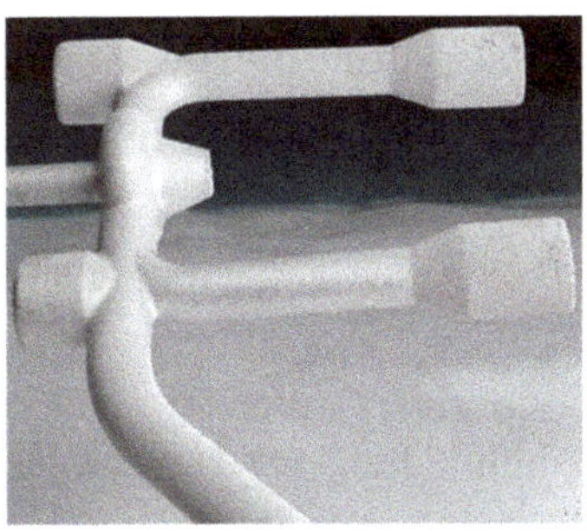

Additional study focused on the comparison between pure magnesium alloys of HA coated and uncoated, as well as the comparison of different cutting geometries between flat and cubic shapes. The report presents that uncoated shapes are influenced by their process production, but the coated version basically decreases the corrosion rate and minor changes are presented [Figure 7].

Figure 7

Comparison between Uncoated and coated PEO Corrosion rate (from EIS).

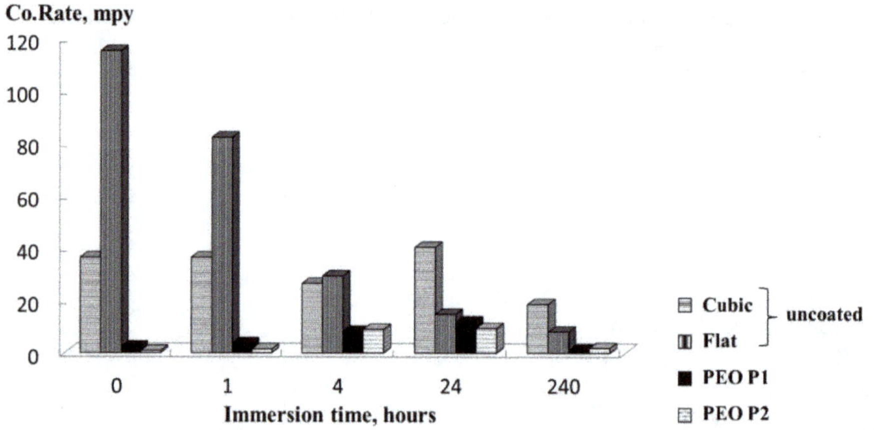

CONCLUSIONS

1. A TiO_2-based coating containing silver particles was successfully deposited on titanium medical grade alloy.
2. This Antimicrobial coating may well be a solution to prevent biofilm formation and could be used on all kind of titanium-based implants especially where high infection risks exist.
3. No silver particles were detected on the biopsies sampled after implantation.
4. No meaningful interfacial cellular, subcellular and matrix changes were observed in either of the silver coated samples.
5. Effective tailoring of corrosion by CaP-PEO upgraded coating for W4 magnesium alloy led to a reduction of corrosion by up to 90%.
6. The results lead to the conclusion that in order to effectively tailor and control the biodegradation of advanced bio-active titanium and magnesium implants, the application of PEO innovative coatings is a very promising method.

REFERENCES

1. Eliezer A., Witte F., "Corrosion behavior of magnesium alloys in biomedical environments", *Journal of Advanced Materials Research*, Vol. 95, 17-22. (2010).
2. Gasqueres C., Schneider G., Nusko R., Maier G., Dingeldein E., Eliezer A., "Innovative antibacterial coating by anodic spark deposition", *Journal of Surface & Coatings Technology*, 206 (2012), 3410-3414.

Paper Number:
C2017-09395

Controlling the Degradation Profile of Mg Biomedical Devices by Alloy Design and Thermomechanical Processing

Stephen LeBeau
nanoMAG

Charles Sfeir
University of Pittsburgh

Raymond Decker
nanoMAG

Boyce Collins
North Carolina A & T University

Abstract

Magnesium (Mg) alloys are gaining interest for biodegradable medical implant devices due to a good combination of mechanical properties and biocompatibility. Nevertheless, the fast degradation rates of Mg and its biocompatible alloys in the aggressive physiological environment impose limitations on their clinical applications. This necessitates the development of Mg based implants with controlled degradation rates to match the kinetics of the bone and tissue healing process and to avoid any complications or issues that might negatively impact surrounding tissues. The current study presents alloy design and thermomechanical processing to optimize the mechanical and biological properties of a new proprietary Mg based alloy. Its corrosion profiles have been evaluated by a combination of *in vitro* and *in vivo* experimental studies. The corrosion rates of laboratory samples and prototype devices have been examined via long term immersion studies by measuring the cumulative amount of hydrogen (H_2) that is emitted by samples. The cumulative H_2 measurements have a direct correlation to the mass loss that the Mg alloy samples undergo during the duration of the tests. The results of the current *in vitro* corrosion studies are compared to 52 week small animal studies to develop predictive models for designing future biomedical devices.

Keywords: magnesium, alloys, thermomechanical processing, bioabsorbable implants, corrosion

INTRODUCTION

Bone trauma, including fracture and osteoporosis, is a major challenge for biomedical engineering. There are about 6 million bone fractures reported in the US annually with a significant number requiring some type of fixation device to facilitate healing. The majority of fixation devices are made of conventional implantable metals like unalloyed titanium (Ti), Ti alloys or stainless steel. However, a significant portion of these non-degradable implants require secondary removal surgeries which are painful and costly; but also risk infections and further fractures. In addition to the implant being permanent, post surgical complications as a result of local tissue reaction and protrusion have been recorded.

Devices constructed with bioabsorbable polymers, e.g. PLLA/PLGA, have been developed to overcome the current concerns and complications with stainless and Ti. These polymer-based devices have limited utility in load bearing sites. In addition, some of the polymer devices have shown some long term foreign body reactions.

There is a need to develop alternate material-based implants for orthopaedic applications. Magnesium and its alloys are potential alternative candidates for biomedical applications due to their biodegradability, non-toxicity and excellent mechanical properties. Mg alloys have physical and mechanical properties that more closely match those of bone compared to Ti or stainless steel. Unlike other metals, Mg alloys have unique biomechanical properties. Mg is widely available in our bodies as the 4th most abundant element present in the body. Mg^{+2} is biocompatible and osteoinductive in promoting new bone growth.[1]

nanoMAG has developed a proprietary Mg alloy, BioMg[(†)], leveraging microalloying with small multiple alloying additions in preference to larger singular or binary additions. This approach provides: a) improved strength, b) lower potential toxicity c) improved ductility and toughness and d) less corrosion compared to excessive alloying additions and e) therefore controlled releases of hydrogen which the human body can accommodate. Microalloying with multiple elements afforded synergistic strengthening at lower overall alloy contents (<3 wt% combined for all three alloying elements) without exceeding the toxicity limits for each individual species. Zinc (Zn), calcium (Ca) and manganese (Mn) all contribute to increased mechanical strength by solid solution and precipitation/ordering mechanisms.[2-17] Mg and the 3 elements are essential in the body a) Mg, Zn and Mn in enzyme mechanisms, b) Ca in skeleton structure and cell functions and c) Mn to mitigate osteoporosis, diabetes mellitus and atherosclerosis. This approach was adopted for design of the new magnesium alloy composition which was evaluated for biodegradability by the *in vitro* and *in vivo* tests described below.[18]

EXPERIMENTAL PROCEDURE AND RESULTS

In vitro Testing via Hydrogen Evolution Methods

There are several commonly used *in vitro* tests, from simple mass loss measurements to more complex electrochemical methods that can be used to measure the biocorrosion rates of magnesium based alloys. Recent critical reviews[19, 20] have assessed the relative merits of each test methodology along with attempts to develop a correlation between *in vitro* and *in vivo* observations. The test methods are divided into two distinct categories: (a) unpolarized and (b) polarized. The electrochemical methods, including potentiodynamic polarization and electrochemical impedance spectroscopy (EIS) have the distinct advantage of providing insight into the corrosion mechanisms involved including the determination of the anodic/cathodic control of the reactions that are occurring. EIS is particularly useful for examining the formation and corrosion reactions of the surface layers on alloy specimens and is particularly useful in the development of surface protective coatings.

For the purposes of screening candidate alloy compositions for use in orthopaedic implants as well as optimization of the manufacturing processing methods for producing medical devices, the authors selected the hydrogen (H_2) evolution method for measuring the biocorrosion of experimental alloys. The advantages of the H_2 evolution methods, examined in detail in earlier publications include: a) setup/sample preparation is easy, b) real time measurement of corrosion over longer time periods, c) the amount of hydrogen measured is directly related to the amount of dissolved magnesium, d) eliminates issues with the corrosion product affecting corrosion measurements observed in standard mass loss studies and e) low cost.[21,22]

The corrosion testing apparatus is shown in Figure 1. The system consists of a 50 gallon aquarium tank that is fitted with a feedback loop controlled heating system to maintain 37°C operating temperature of a synthetic body fluid (SBF) solution (including

† Registered trademark of nanoMAG, LLC.

Figure 1

(a) Overview of corrosion tank displaying system for collection and measurement of H_2 gas evolved for each individual specimen (b) Poly mesh suspension system provides uniform exposure of samples to SBF.

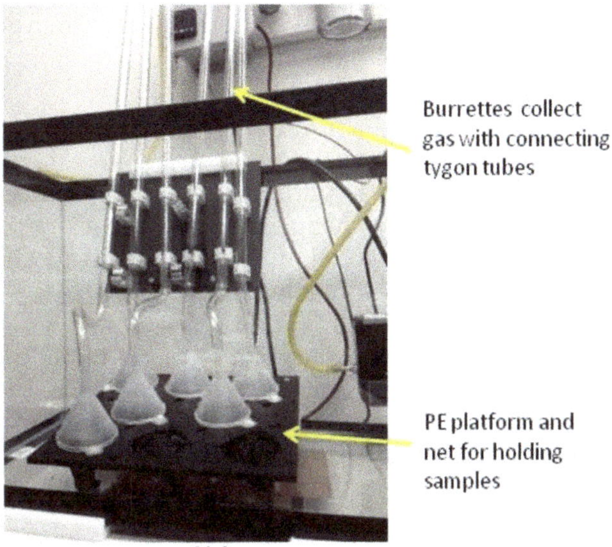

1(a).

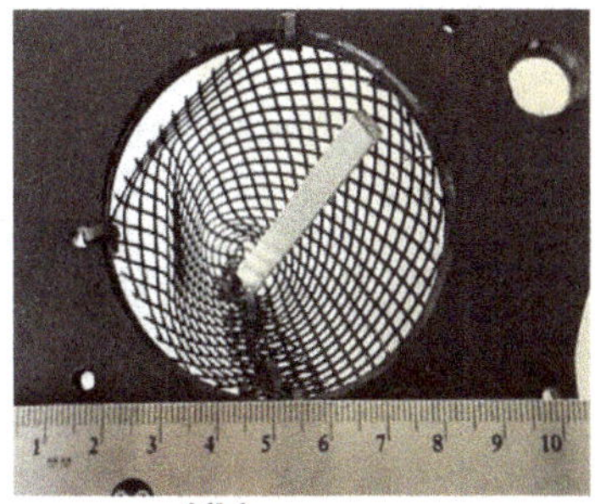

1(b).

a recirculation pump, particle filter and UV filter to maintain the SBF solution quality). The test specimens (up to 18 samples can be evaluated at one time) are suspended in a cone shaped poly mesh to allow consistent exposure of the entire surface of the specimen to the circulating fluid (Figure 1b). Each individual specimen holder is covered with an inverted cone (75 ml) that is plumbed directly into a graduated 100 ml burette to measure the H_2 generated during the biocorrosion testing. The poly mesh specimen containers and inverted cones are supported by a polyethylene plate with holes cut into the plates for each sample location. Insulation (2 inch thick styrene) is attached to the exterior sides and top of the tank for thermal stability. Polyethylene sheet is used to cover the tank to prevent evaporation of the solution and to provide an additional thermal barrier for the tank.

These *in vitro* tests were run at 37°C and pH 7.4 in SBF composed of phosphate buffered saline solution. A fresh batch of SBF was prepared in 30 gallon quantities with the following chemical additions (Table 1) made in 100°C preheated ADI water that was then cooled down to 37°C and the pH was measured and adjusted as necessary to 7.4.

Table 1

Chemical makeup of SBF used for current study - 30 gallon batch.

Chemical Name	Formula	Amount(grams)
Sodium Chloride	NaCl	908.8
Potassium Chloride	KCi	22.72
Sodium Phosphate	Na_2HPO_4	163.58
Potassium Phosphate	KH_2PO_4	27.26

Each burette was filled completely with SBF solution prior to the start of the test and then attached to the funnel/tubing above the specimen. Hydrogen generated by the sample displaces the solution in each burette allowing a direct measurement to be made for each specimen on a daily basis. The temperature of the SBF bath and pH were recorded daily along with the measurement of the cumulative H_2 generated by each individual specimen. Daily H_2 evolution was recorded as a measure of Mg corrosion due to the following reaction:

(1)

$$Mg(s) + 2H_2O(aq) \rightarrow Mg(OH)_2(s) + H_2(gas)$$

Thus, the evolution of 1 mole of H_2 gas (22.4 liters) directly corresponds to the dissolution of 1 mole of Mg (24.31 grams). For measurements made on the current test system normally in units of milliliters of hydrogen, 1.0 ml of H_2 is equivalent to 1.085 mg of magnesium that is dissolved. Unlike mass loss immersion testing systems, the H_2 system is not affected by the corrosion products (which may in fact lead to a weight gain in samples if the corrosion products are not removed prior to measurements).[19] The primary advantage of the H_2 evolution system is the ability to take measurements at multiple time points throughout the test, allowing the analysis of the changes in corrosion rate occurring over the time duration of the experiment.

Experimental variables that have to be managed carefully during hydrogen evolution tests include: SBF bath temperature, pH of the solution, the volume of SBF solution to specimen surface area (which could lead to local increases in pH levels if the solution is too low in volume relative to the specimens) and insuring that all of the surfaces of the specimens are exposed to the SBF solution. With the daily measurements being used for the current testing protocol and the poly mesh suspended design for holding specimens; these concerns have been addressed in the current study. If the bath pH level exceeds 7.8, the entire solution is discarded and replaced with fresh solution.

Finally, the volume of H_2 gas generated per mole is governed by the ideal gas law given by:

(2)

$$PV=nRT$$

where P is the pressure, V is the volume, n is the amount of gas in moles, R is the ideal gas constant and T is the temperature (K). The potential variance caused by different atmospheric pressures can be significant. For example, an experiment performed at an elevation of 2000 m would evolve almost 30% more volume of H_2 than when performed at sea level.

A rectangular beam specimen geometry was chosen, 6.8 cm X 0.6 cm cross section and 0.3 cm thick (Figure 2). This geometry allows the corrosion rate to be measured over various time points and then a three point compression bend test can be performed to measure the mechanical degradation profile after extraction from the tank. The corrosion system will also accept other geometries including manufactured biomedical devices. Rectangular samples for *in vitro* corrosion tests were prepared by machining to the finished dimensions followed by sanding on 400 grit paper, passivation treatment (an alkaline wash, water rinse, and mild hydrochloric acid passivation treatment followed by rinsing in distilled water, rinsing in isopropyl alcohol and forced air drying.

Figure 2

Typical sample geometries tested in the corrosion system; top to bottom; rectangular beam for SBF testing and 3 point bending; 7 mm diameter ACL screw and 3 mm diameter suture anchor.

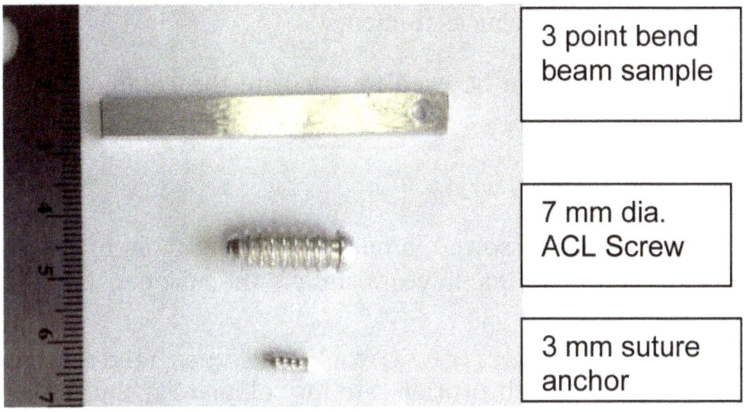

Figure 3

Hydrogen Evolution Comparison of Experimental alloy with Commercial Alloys.

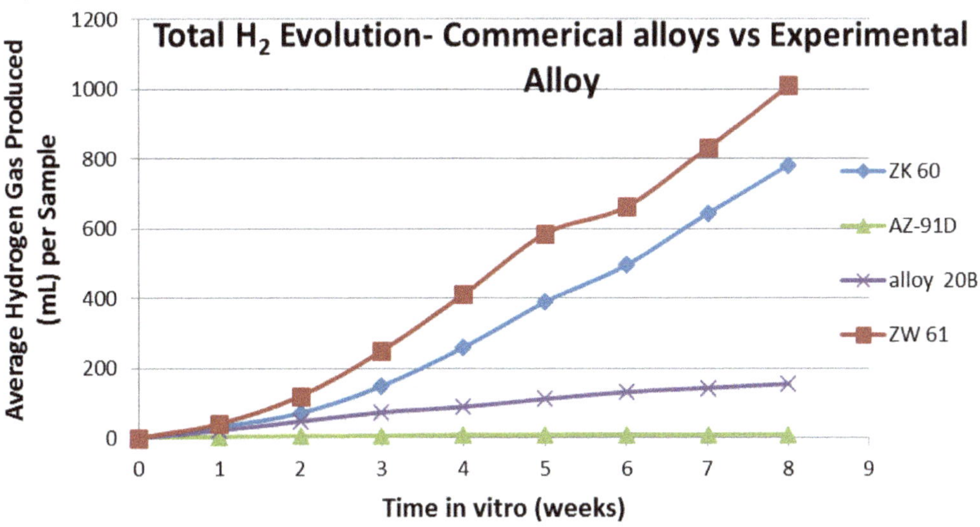

Initial comparison testing of experimental alloy compositions was performed over an 8 week test period (Figure 3). The cumulative total H_2 evolution observed over 8 weeks ranged from a low of 10.4 ml (AZ-91D) to a high of 1009 ml (ZW-61). The displayed curves are average values obtained from three replicate samples of each alloy composition. Alloy 20-B is an early experimental alloy composition that was being evaluated for possible use in orthopedic implants. Examination of the curves reveals the following trends for the hydrogen evolution:

1. The effective corrosion rate can vary considerably over the duration of a test.
2. In as little as three weeks, the respective long term absorption profiles for each alloy are predicted with a high degree of certainty.
3. The H_2 evolution method can provide comparative analysis of candidate alloys in a reasonable time frame with simple measurements.

The H_2 evolution values in milliliters can be used to calculate the commonly used corrosion rate, CR, by the formula;

(3)

$$CR = W/At\rho$$

where W = the weight of magnesium dissolved in milligrams (1.085 X ml of H_2), A = surface area of the specimen (mm^2), t = time in years and ρ = the bulk density of the magnesium alloy(mg/mm^3).

The respective measured biocorrosion rates (Table 2) would indicate that the commercial alloy AZ-91D may have too slow an absorption rate for commercial applications, whereas the ZK-60 and ZW-61 alloys examined indicate an absorption rate that may be too accelerated for implant applications. The authors have developed a new proprietary alloy composition that would provide a stable absorption profile and mechanical degradation through the initial healing process; followed by a stable absorption until final absorption with no negative effects on the surrounding tissues. The target for total absorption for *in vivo* implants is 12-18 months post surgery with variations expected based on specimen geometries and the anatomical location in the body.

Alloy Design for Optimum Strength and Absorption Profiles

A. *In vitro* Testing

Experimental Mg-Zn-Ca-Mn alloys were prepared by melting under a 5% blend of SF_6 with Argon and casting into steel molds. Such cast forms were homogenized, warm rolled and heat treated in preparation for *in vitro* corrosion testing. After optimization of the composition, a commercial production heat (100 kg quantity) was produced for both *in vitro* and *in vivo* corrosion evaluation and for mechanical testing. Bend strength was tested on rectangular samples, 6.8 cm X 0.6 cm cross section and 0.3 cm thick by 3 point bending at a strain rate of 0.5 inch/min.[27]

The effect of alloying elements on *in vitro* corrosion is seen in Table 3. Corrosion was increased and retained strength decreased with Zn above 2% and Ca at 0.6%. High Zn led to excess Mg_2Zn particles, anodic to the matrix and accelerating corrosion. High Ca

Table 2

Calculated Corrosion Rates for Several Mg Alloys at Two Stages of H_2 Evolution Testing.

Alloy grade	CR (mm/yr) 0 - 4 weeks	CR (mm/yr) 4-8 weeks
AZ-91D	0.05	0.01
Alloy 20B	0.58	0.42
ZK-60	1.67	3.37
ZW 61	2.65	3.86

produced Mg_2Ca and/or $Ca_2Mg_6Zn_3$ particles, also detrimental to corrosion. Optimum response of experimental alloys in SBF was at Mg-1Zn-0.3Ca-0.5Mn. This micro alloyed response in SBF was confirmed by scale-up to the commercial heat of the alloy which outperformed the experimental heats. Producing alloys on a larger commercial scale with proper use of cover gas during melting and cropping of cast billets to remove any shrinkage areas and surface contaminants, reduces the likelihood of entrapment of oxides or segregation observed in small laboratory batches of 1-2 kg. This refinement in the microstructure supports the observations on improving corrosion resistance and better mechanical properties.

To verify the reproducibility of *in vitro* degradation rate of the Mg-Zn-Ca-Mn alloy derived from processing of various geometries and devices, experimental bend samples were compared to craniomaxillofacial (CMF) fracture fixation plates and CMF screws in Table 4. The three geometric forms had comparable response in SBF when the hydrogen evolution rates were adjusted to account for the specific surface area of each specimen geometry.

Table 3

Effect of Alloy Content on SBF Corrosion of Mg Alloys.

Alloy Content	% Bend Strength Retained-after 2 weeks in SBF	H_2 Evolution, 2 weeks, ml	H_2 Evolution, 5 weeks, ml
Mg-4Zn-0.3Ca-0.6Mn	75	100	250
Mg-3Zn-0.3Ca-0.5Mn	47	140	-
Mg-2Zn-0.6Ca-0.4Mn	28	120	740
Mg-2Zn-0.3Ca-0.4Mn	73	70	241
Mg-1Zn-0.6Ca-0.2Mn	53	100	200
Mg-1Zn-0.3Ca-0.3Mn	86	75	101
Mg-1Zn-0.3Ca-0.1Mn	-	40	90
Mg-1Zn-0.3Ca-0.5Mn	-	33	56
Commercial Alloy	90	12	56

Table 4

Effect of Geometry of Commercial Alloy on *in vitro* Corrosion Rate.

Geometry	H2 (ml) 14 days	Surface area (cm^2)	CR, $ml/cm^2/day$
Bend Test Bar	14.2	12.47	0.08
CMF Screw	2.9	2.19	0.09
CMF Plate	12.4	8.9	0.10

Figure 4

Suture Screw Design (3 mm dia. by 5 mm long) for Implants (both Magnesium alloy and PLGA machined to same geometry).

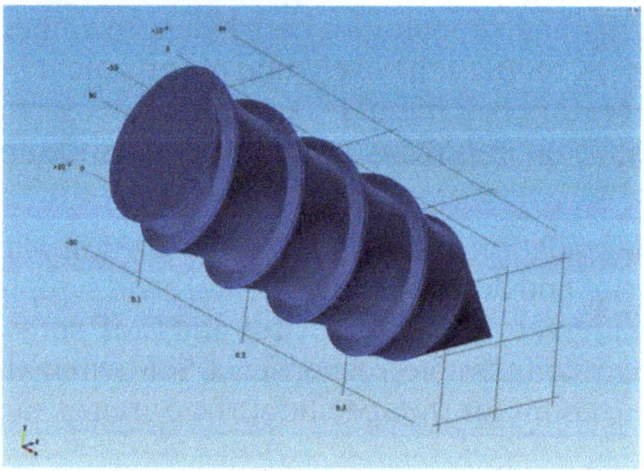

B. *In vivo* Testing

Initial small animal tests on the bioabsorbable Mg based alloy have been conducted at a university research facility. Side by side femoral implants of the Mg based alloy with comparable control samples of a PLGA-based bioresorbable polymer were placed in 12 rabbits for time points ranging from 2 weeks to 52 weeks. After access to the knee joint was obtained using osteotomy, an 8 mm deep hole was drilled through the cartilage into the cancellous part of the lateral femur condyle. Then implants (3 mm in diameter by 5 mm in height), see Figure 4 below, were inserted into the drilled holes of the knees by a press fit technique. A 2.7 mm diameter drill bit size was used for a 3 mm diameter implant to achieve the press fit. Animals were sacrificed at 2, 4, 12, 24, 36 and 52 weeks (n=12) after surgery with two animals harvested at each time point.

Harvested specimens were evaluated by a combination of micro CT and histology examinations. Before sample retrieval, the animals were euthanized by an intravenous overdose of 2 ml/4.5 kg dose of 240 mg/ml pentobarbital after sedation. Once a pneumothorax has been created, the medial condyles were dissected as a block from the knee joint and placed in neutral buffered formalin (NBF, 10% buffered methanolic formalin at 100% strength) for preservation. The explant samples were imaged in formalin by X-ray computed tomography. Representative X-ray emission parameters of the micro-CT included a voltage of 60 kV and current of 80 μA. Typically, 2000 projections were collected (single scan average = 2) per 360 degree rotation and the 3-D renderings were analyzed using analytical software. Micro CT allows the analysis of the remaining volume of the embedded implanted material non-destructively while preserving the embedded implants for subsequent histology.

After micro CT, the condyles were fixed in 3.7% commercial formalin for 7 days at 4°C. Consequently, the non-decalcified samples were embedded in plastic and five micrometer sections were cut and processed. The Mg based alloy embedded implants were prepared with two stains a) Masson's Trichrome which stains the bone blue and connective tissue pink to red and b) Sanderson's Rapid Bone Stain which stains the bone purple. Masson's Trichrome does not distinguish between old and new bone but Sanderson's does. The rapid bone stain is a fabulous cellular stain which provides distinct contrast as seen in the bottom left images in Figure 5 for the samples extracted

Figure 5

Histology slides for 12 week post surgery Mg based alloy implants (note presence of bone in intimate contact with the Mg alloy implant).

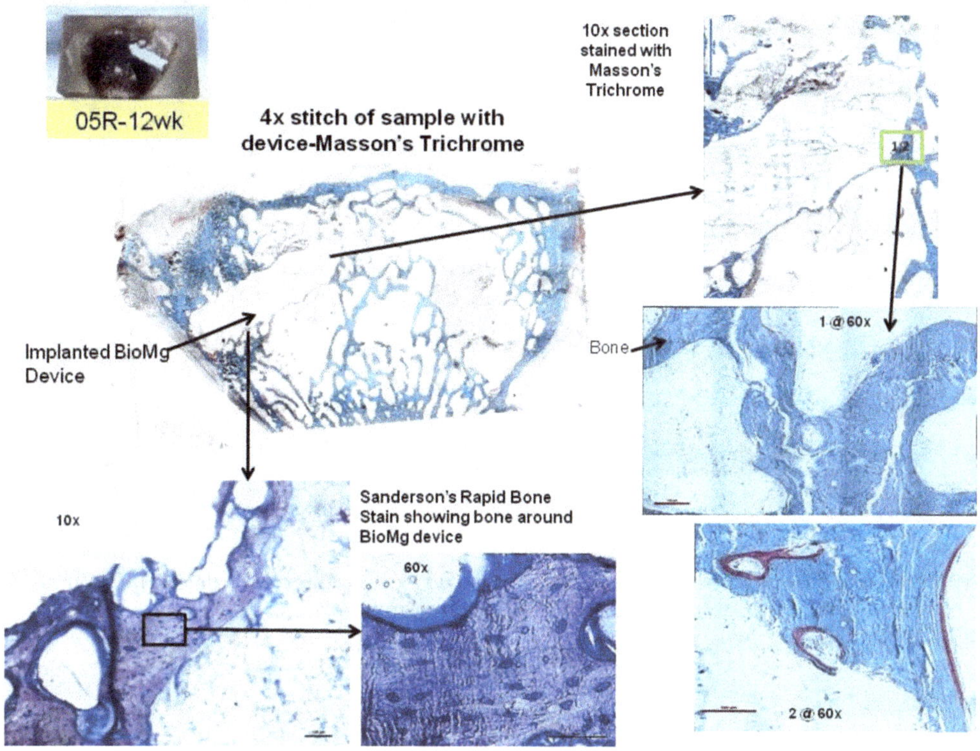

12 weeks post surgery. The two sets of images were taken in what was considered new bone, along the device interface, away from the native bone. This is the first timepoint when bone bridging was observed along most of the Mg based alloy interface.

Micro-CT Studies

By utilizing software to analyze various sections of the implants the CT imaging was co-localized with histology. Upon generation of histology data, the 3-D rendered volume was oriented using the details of the stained tissue slice so that a virtual slice of CT data could be compared almost directly with the histology. In this way, the CT imaging became more informative as shades of grey become more revealing. An example of this technique is shown in Figure 6. The cancellous bone is similarly patterned in both images.

Examination of micro-CT images alone raised concerns about suspicious areas of the images that are of darker contrast suggesting these areas may represent gas pockets that are surrounding the Mg alloy implants during the bioabsorption process. Comparison of the same areas displayed on the histology images taken from the same explants suggest these varying levels of contrast in the CT images may in fact be misinterpreted as gas pockets and may simply be areas of tissue of lower density. Future animal studies on bioabsorbable Mg alloy implants that employ micro-CT imaging techniques should also employ alternate imaging methods to cross reference the same areas of implants.

Figure 6

Co-localized data: histology (left) and X-ray CT (right) for week 24 explants.

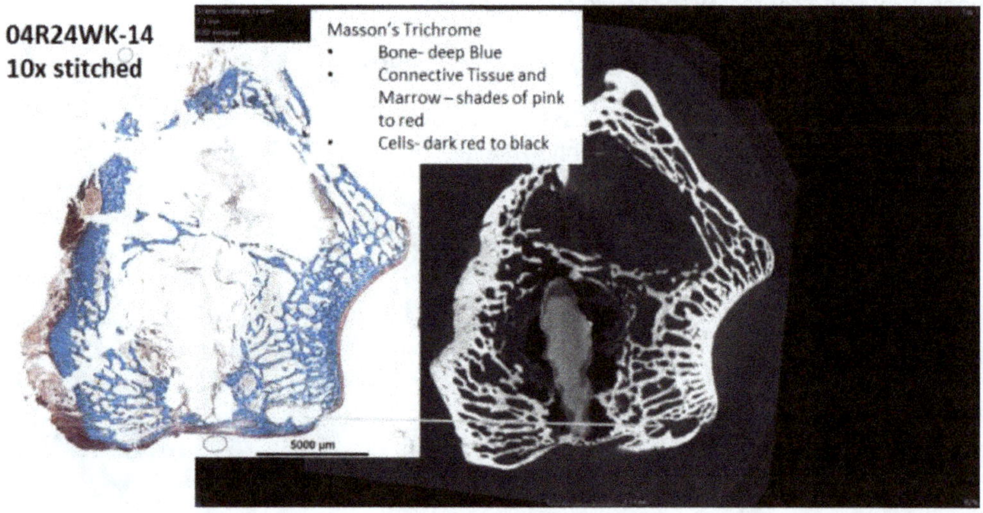

Figure 7

Graph of estimated volume loss (+/- 10%) vs. *in vivo* exposure from CT data. The volume is based on grayscale segmentation and Gaussian fits to data.

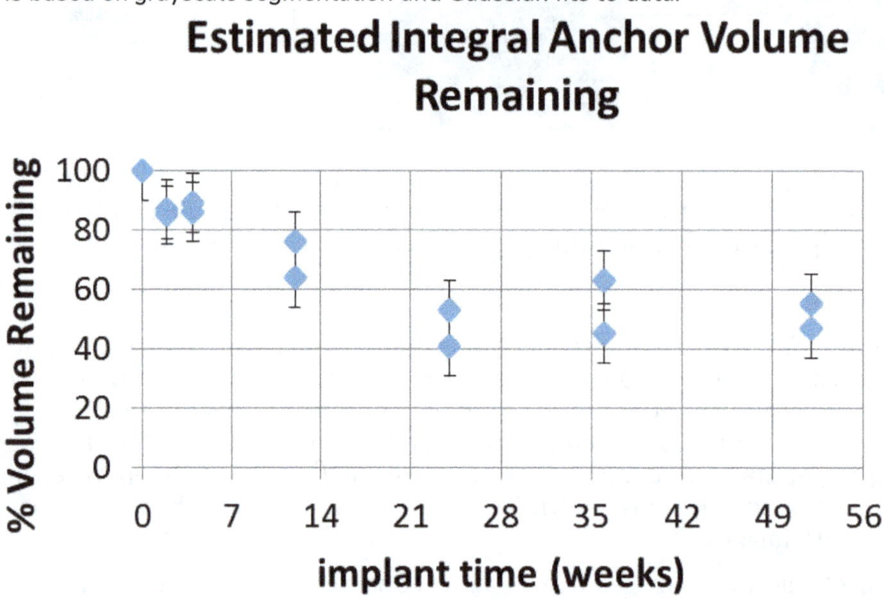

Multiple CT scans over several time points can be used to forecast the absorption rates of the Mg implants and can be used to develop predictive models of the bioabsorption behavior. The graph presented in Figure 7 shows a forecast of the qualitative volume of the implanted screw absorbed over time using a 3-D software tool package. This current forecast is based on limited data and only two samples per each time point. Utilizing this data trend and corrosion modeling a dissolution rate of ~0.2 mm/yr was estimated for the current implant geometry embedded in the femoral area of the

Figure 8

52 week histology displaying contact between new bone and Mg alloy implant.

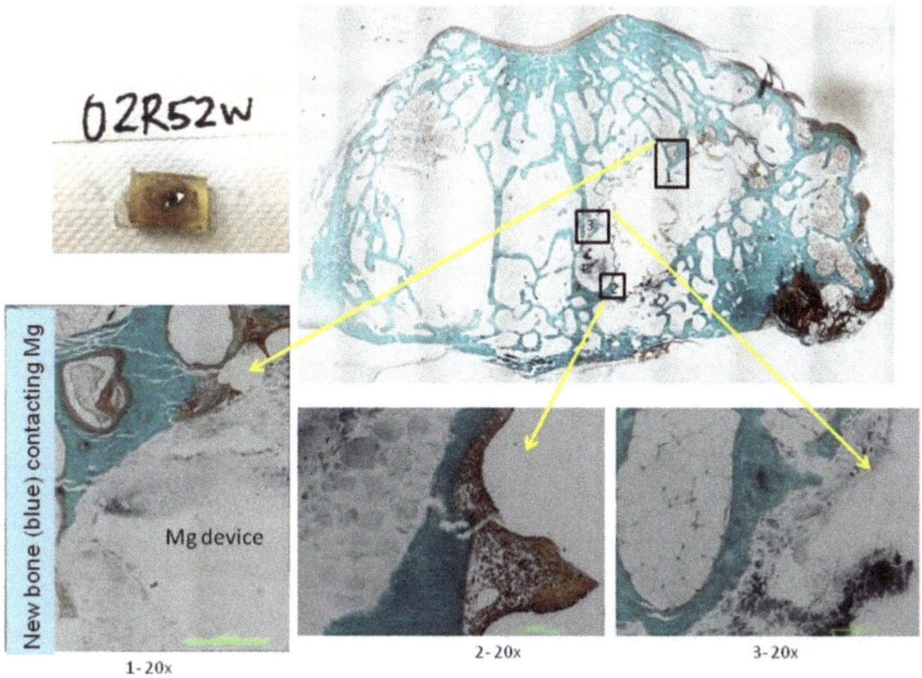

rabbits. Comparison examinations of *in vitro* studies with *in vivo* studies are proposed in the future rounds of large animal testing to continue the software optimization for micro CT examinations to develop *in vitro* – *in vivo* correlations with varying implant geometries and *in vivo* implantation sites.

The histology data for the Mg alloy implant samples after 52 week post surgery (Figure 8) confirms the implant has experienced approximately 50 volume % absorption over the 52 weeks. From the micro CT data, the equivalent corrosion rate (mm/year) can be estimated by the following formula:

(4)

$$CR = \Delta V / At$$

where CR= corrosion rate (mm/year), delta V is % volume reduction times the original volume of the 3 mm suture anchor device (33.053 mm^3), A is the original surface area of the device (70.0648 $mm^{2)}$, and t is the time in years. The estimated corrosion rate

Table 5

Variation of estimated Corrosion Rates at Different Stages of *in vivo* testing.

Time interval of in vivo test	Estimated CR (mm/yr) based on micro-CT data
0-12 weeks	0.61
12-36 weeks	0.16
36 - 52 weeks	0.05

Figure 9

SEM of residual implant after 52 weeks in vivo, with corrosion reaction layer and encapsulating new bone.

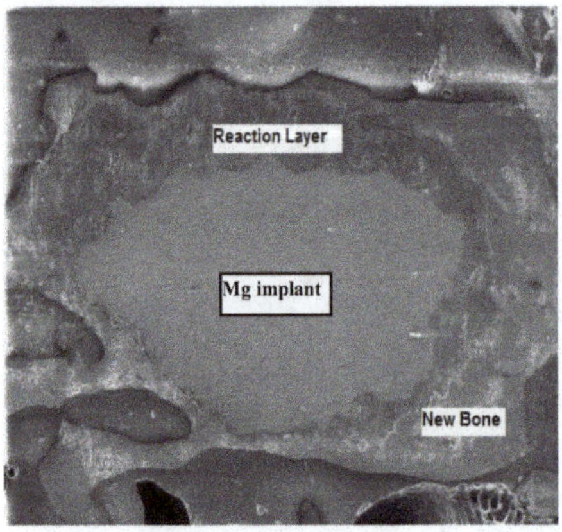

Figure 10

Magnesium (Mg) Map concentrated in residual implant.

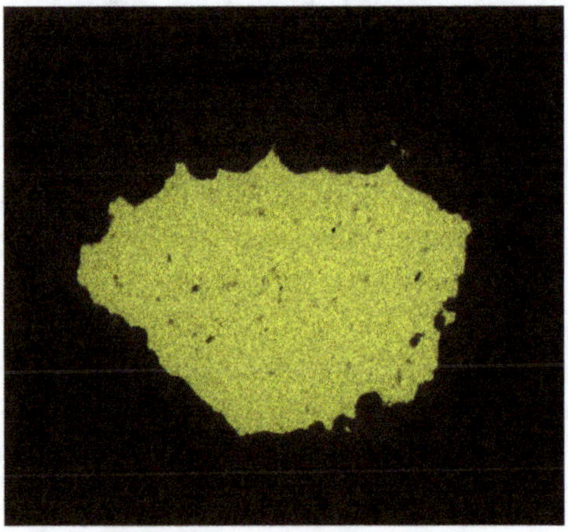

over the duration of the *in vitro* test based on the above formula is 0.23 mm/yr. If you examine the date more carefully, the corrosion rate is not linear over the entire time of the testing as shown in estimated corrosion rates at different time intervals of the *in vivo* tests (Table 5).

As seen in Figure 5, new bone coverage of the Mg alloy implanted screw was evident as soon as 12 weeks *in vivo*. This coverage by new bone progressed through 52 weeks when the residual implant was encompassed in a corrosion reaction layer that was, in turn, being replaced by new bone (see Figure 9).

By Scanning Electron Microscopy (SEM) and Energy Dispersive Spectroscopy (EDS) imaging and linear scans, the alloying elements were located in a) the residual implant, b) a transition corrosion layer and c) in new bone that encapsulated and replaced the implant and corrosion layer. The SEM images for the elemental distribution of the major alloying constituents in Figures 9-13. Quantitative measurements of alloying contents in the transition corrosion layer and new bone are included in Table 6. In

Figure 11

Calcium (Ca) Map displaying incorporation of calcium in the transition layer between new bone and residual.

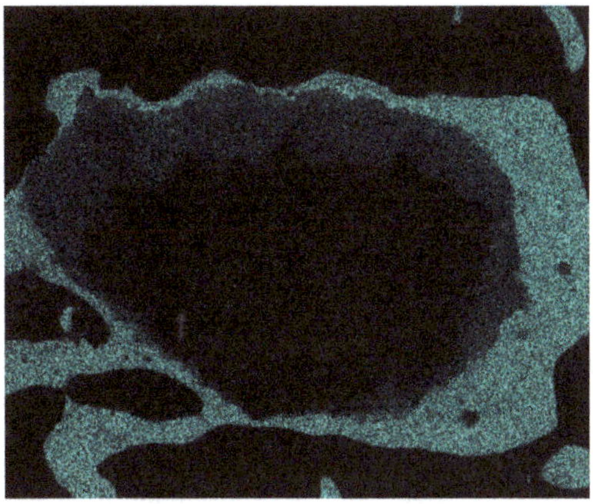

Figure 12

Phosphorous (P) Map with behavior similar to Calcium.

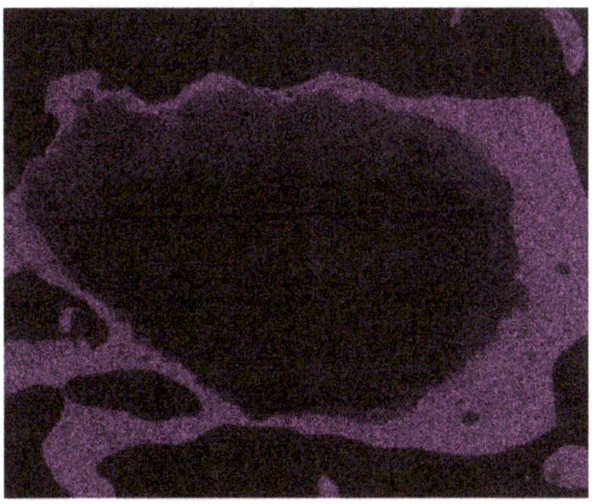

Figure 13

Zinc (Zn) Map with possible segregation into precipitates in transition layer.

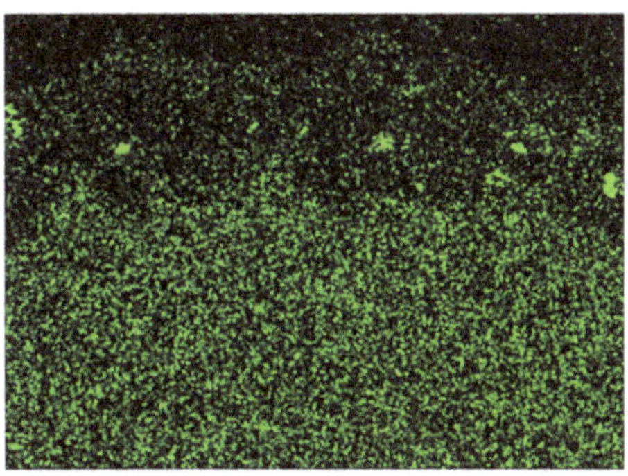

concert with the literature and the role in corrosion, Zn and Mn were found in the transition corrosion layer; in the case of Zn segregated in particles in the transition layer (Figure 13). Mg, Zn, Ca, P, O, and Mn were found alloyed in the new bone, probably related to their osteoinductivity.

DISCUSSION

In vitro corrosion tests are valuable in approximating the effects of microalloying design and in selecting the nominal composition of new bioabsorbable alloys being developed for use in orthopedic medical implants. Since *in vitro* testing is much less costly than animal testing and since alloying trends can be discerned in a matter of 2 weeks in SBF vs. a year in animals, *in vitro* SBF testing has real utility. The subsequent *in vivo* results observed in the current study displayed bioabsorption profiles that were consistent with the predictions from SBF *in vitro* tests.

Published results for comparison of *in vitro* to *in vivo* rates for Mg alloys have reported *in vitro* degradation rates have typically ranged from 1 to 4 times faster than *in vivo* rates. One possible explanation for the observed lower rates *in vivo* is the lower concentration of chloride ions in blood plasma and bone. As demonstrated by the current study, short time measurements of both *in vitro* and *in vivo* rates can be substantially different than those values obtained based on longer time intervals (i.e.> 30 days). The *in vitro* bioabsorption rates estimated based on the micro-CT measurements were initially higher (0.61 mm/yr for the first 12 weeks) followed by significantly lower rates (0.16 mm/yr for 12-36 weeks and 0.05 mm/yr for 36 to 52 weeks). The observations made on the same time intervals by histology and micro-CT exhibited the encapsulation of the bioabsorbable implants by a layer of newly formed bone with the initial formation observed as early as 12 weeks. These observations on the encapsulation of the implants by new tissue structures may explain the reduction in corrosion rates seen at the later time points.

Samples that are subjected to *in vitro* tests quite frequently display initially higher biocorrosion rates until a surface protective layer is observed on the surface of the samples. These corrosion products can also coat the sample surface and reduce the observed biocorrosion rates, particularly in tests that are conducted in static fluid conditions.

Table 6

SEM linear scan results on Mg alloy implant after 52 weeks *in vivo* in rabbit.

Element	% in Alloy	% in Transition Layer	% in New Bone
Mg	97.9	23-30	1.4-6.6
Zn	1.3	1.0- 1.7	0.22 - 0.31
Ca	0.4	11 - 15	38-41
Mn	0.4	0.2-0.5	0.08-0.14
P	-	4-10	18-19
0	-	49-53	37-40

The reported differences in corrosion behavior *in vitro* and *in vivo* can be attributed in part to the difficulties in mimicking the complex physiological conditions *in vitro*. Lack of detailed information and the highly variable methodologies employed in previous studies limit the ability to draw comparisons of the corrosion behavior. The use of standardized methods or common protocols for measuring biocorrosion rates and more detailed reporting on the experimental procedures used will help develop our understanding of the biocorrosion behavior of magnesium alloys. Research technologists are encouraged to provide more detailed experimental parameters in their published work and work to develop standardized methods to contribute to the overall commercial development of bioabsorbable alloys.

CONCLUSIONS

1. *In vitro* testing can be a very effective screening tool in the alloy design of bioabsorbable Mg alloys.
2. Measured rates of biocorrosion rates are generally higher *in vitro* but with careful experimental methods can be effective for providing trends on observed *in vivo* rates.
3. The method of hydrogen evolution measurement can be a cost effective and efficient process for screening candidate's alloys and manufacturing processing providing very consistent comparative data on biocorrosion rates over longer time intervals.
4. Experimental approaches that incorporate a multitude of methodologies; polarized vs non-polarized for *in vitro* testing and a combination of histology and micro-CT for *in vivo* are essential to develop systematic correlations for magnesium alloy biocorrosion.
5. A new bioabsorbable Magnesium based alloy that displays the target bioabsorption rates for use in orthopedic implants has been developed and is ongoing additional pre-clinical studies for FDA submission. The development time for producing this new alloy was substantially shortened by utilizing the corrosion experimental methods described in this manuscript.

ACKNOWLEDGEMENTS

This work was supported by the NSF Engineering Research Center for Revolutionizing Metallic Biomaterials (ERC-RMB) based at the North Carolina State A & T University, under sponsorship of NSF STTR IIB Project No. 0847198. The authors also want to acknowledge the technical contributions of Elizabeth Perepezko of Zimmer Biomet for her input on testing protocols for both *in vitro* and *in vivo* methods.

REFERENCES

1. Zheng, Y., *Magnesium Alloys as Degradable Biomaterials*, CRC Press (2016), ISBN-13: 978-1-4665-9804-1.
2. Kallyanashis P., Lee P. B.Y., Abueva C., Kim B., Choi H., Bae S., Lee B. T., "*In vivo* evaluation of injectable calcium phosphate cement composed of Zn-and Si-incorporated β-tricalcium phosphate and monocalcium phosphate monohydrate for a critical sized defect of the rabbit femoral condyle", *J. Biomedical Materials Research B. Applied Biomaterials*, 2016, (in press).

3. Moreno-Eutimio M., "Potent Anti-inflammatory Activity of Carbohydrate Polymer of Zinc," *Biomed Res Int*, 2014, p.8.
4. Chou A., LeGoros R., Chen Z., "Anti-bacterial Effect of Zinc Phosphate on Mineralized Bone Regeneration", *Implant Dentistry*, 2007, 16, p.89.
5. Yang F., Dong W., He F., Wang X., Zhao S., Yang G., "Osteoblast response to porous Ti surfaces coated with zinc-substituted hypoxyapatite", *Oral Surg Oral Med Oral Pathol Oral Radiol*, 2012, 113, p. 313.
6. Zakiyuddin A., Lee K., "Effect of small addition of zinc and manganese to Mg-Ca based alloys on degradation behavior in physiological media", *J. Alloys and Compounds*, 629 (2015), p. 274.
7. Kwak H. and Chaudhuri S., "Cationic doping of MgO surfaces to build corrosion protection in Mg alloys", *J. Alloys and Compounds*, 509 (2011), p. 8189.
8. Tong L., Zheng M., Xu S., Kamadu S., Du Y., Hu X., Wu K., Gan W., Brokmeier H., Wang G., Li X., "Effect of Mn Addition on microstructure, texture and properties of Mg-Zn-Ca Alloy", *Materials Science and Engineering* A, 528 (2011), p. 3741.
9. Yasi S., Hector L., Trinkle D., "First-principles data for solid-solution hardening of magnesium: from geometry and chemistry to properties", *Acta Materialia*, 58 (2010), p. 5704).
10. Liu Y-T., Kung K-C., Lee T-M., Lui T-S., "Enhancing biological properties of porous coatings through the incorporation of manganese", *J. Alloys and Compounds*, 581 (2013), p. 459.
11. Bae Y-J. and Kim M-H., "Manganese Supplementation Improves Mineral Density of the Spine and Femur and Serum Osteocalcin in Rats", *Biol.Trace Elem. Res.*, 124 (2008), p. 28.
12. Sima F., Socol G., Axente E., Mihailescu L., Zdrentu L., Petrescu S., Mayer I., "Biocompatible and bioactive coatings of Mn^{2+}-doped β-tricalcium phosphate synthesized by pulsed laser deposition", *Applied Surface Science*, 254 (2007), p. 1155.
13. Bigi A., Bracci B., Cuisinier F., Elkaim R., Fini M., Mayer I., Mihailescu I., Socol G., Sturba L., Torricelli P., "Human osteoblast response to pulsed laser deposited calcium phosphate coatings", *Biomaterials*, 26 (2005), p.2381.
14. Bracci B., Torricelli T., Panzavolta S., Boanini E., Giardino R., Bigi A., "Effect of Mg^{2+}, Sr^{2+}, and Mn^{2+} on the chemico-physical and in vitro biological properties of calcium phosphate biomimetic coatings", *J. Inorganic Biochemistry*, 103 (2009), p. 1666.
15. Aeseth J., Boivin G., Andersen O., "Osteoporosis and trace elements – An Overview", *J. Trace Elements in Medicine and Biology*, 26 (2012), p. 149.
16. Chesnick I., Centeno J., Todorov T., Koenig A., Potter K., "Spatial Mapping of mineralization with manganese-enhanced magnetic resonance imaging", *Bone*, 48 (2011), p. 1194.
17. Yoshizawa S., Brown A., Barchowsky A., Sfeir C., "Magnesium ion stimulation of bone marrow stromal cells enhances osteogenic activity, simulating the effect of magnesium alloy degradation", *Acta Biomateriala*, 10(2014), p. 2842.
18. Decker R., LeBeau S., Young S., "High Strength and Bio-absorbable Magnesium Alloys", *National Science Foundation Contract* 0847198 *and related International Patent Application* PCT 2014/030477 (BioMg® 250).
19. Sanchez A.H.M., Luthringer B.J.C., Feyeraband F., Willumeit R., "Mg and Mg alloys: How comparable are in vitro and in vivo corrosion rates? A review." *Acta Biomaterialia*, (2014) http://dx.doi.org/10.1016/jactbio.2014.11.048.

20. Kirkland N.T., Birbills N., Staiger M.P., “Assessing the corrosion of biodegradable magnesium implants: A critical review of current methodologies and their limitations.” *Acta Biomateriala*, 8 (2012) 925-936.
21. Song G., Atrens A., St John D., “An hydrogen evolution method for the estimation of the corrosion rate of magnesium alloys.”, “Magnesium Technology Symposium: 2001 New Orleans; Minerals, Metals and Materials Society, p. 255 – 262. JN Hyrn, Editor.
22. ASTM E390, "*Standard Test Methods for Bend Testing of Material for Ductility*", ASTM International 2009.

Paper Number:
C2017-09537

Electrochemical Studies of Titanium-Boron Alloys in Physiological Solutions

S. McCarthy
California State Polytechnic University

R. Rodriguez
California State Polytechnic University

K. Robles
California State Polytechnic University

J. Fly
California State Polytechnic University

J. Medina
California State Polytechnic University

V. A. Ravi
California State Polytechnic University

L. Nguyen
California State Polytechnic University

Abstract

Modern structural biomedical implants utilize titanium alloys due to their excellent corrosion resistance, mechanical properties and biocompatibility. An important mode of failure with the implant alloys, e.g., UNS R56400 (Ti-6Al-4V; Ti64), is aseptic loosening. This is a phenomenon initiated by the release of particles from the implants, leading to excessive bone erosion. The purpose of this study is to quantitatively compare the corrosion behavior of Ti64 with and without boron addition in various physiological solutions. In this study, these alloys were subjected to cyclic potentiodynamic polarization tests in deaerated Donor Bovine Serum (DBS) and Lactated Ringer's Solution (Ringer's). Comparisons to alloy performance in Phosphate Buffered Saline (PBS) were also made. None of the alloys tested showed signs of breakdown. Additionally, for small amounts of boron additions to Ti64, the passivation potentials decrease.

Keywords: titanium, boron, corrosion, ASTM F2129-15, biomedical implant

INTRODUCTION

Modern structural biomedical implants are made from titanium alloys because of their biocompatibility and favorable corrosion resistance. Currently UNS R56400 (Ti-6Al-4V; Ti64), the most common structural implant alloy, provides 12-15 years of service.[1] As the life expectancy of patients increases, alloys that are longer-lasting would be beneficial for avoiding revision surgery. One of the major causes of implant failures is by aseptic loosening, which is caused by the reaction of the body to the debris produced by implant corrosion and/or wear.[2] The introduction of vanadium ions into the body can also pose complications by inducing an inflammatory response in the surrounding tissue, while aluminum ions can increase the possibility of the development of Alzheimer's upon long-term exposure.[3] Boron is a promising alloying element that has been shown to reduce inflammation, alleviate arthritis, and help with bone growth and maintenance.[4,5] Studies thus far have shown that trace amounts of boron added to Ti64 can improve the corrosion behavior[6-10] of the base alloy along with increases to the strength of the alloy.

EXPERIMENTAL PROCEDURE

The alloys tested were Ti64 with boron contents in 0 to 0.5 wt% range. The alloys were cast as cylinders and were subsequently hot isostatically pressed. Test coupons in the form of discs 13 ± 1 mm (0.51" ± 0.04") diameter and a thickness of 7 ± 2 mm (0.28" ± .08") were machined from the original cylindrical ingots (nominally 30 x 7 cm).

Sample Preparation

The test coupons were ground sequentially from 240 to 800 grit silicon carbide paper and polished using oil-dispersed diamond paste with particle sizes of 6, 3 and 1 µm. The final surface finish was obtained using an aqueous suspension of 0.05 µm alumina. The coupons were then sonicated in both water and acetone as the final preparation step.

Corrosive Media

Table 1 shows the compositions for Phosphate Buffered Saline (PBS) and Lactated Ringer's Solution (Ringer's) that were used for the corrosion tests.

The Donor Bovine Serum (DBS) contains proteins including albumin and12 globulin; bilirubin (iron, cholesterol, triglycerides, glucose) as well as creatinine and uric acid in addition to other constituents including chlorides and bicarbonates. The DBS was diluted to 10 volume% in 18.2 MΩ-cm type 1 reagent water.

Corrosion Tests

The corrosion experiments were conducted using the F2129-15[11] (F2129) test protocol as a guide. A 3-electrode flat cell with a 250 cm^3 capacity was used for corrosion testing. The test solution was heated to 37°C and maintained at a constant temperature with a heating jacket around the flat cell. Deaeration was performed using flowing nitrogen

Table 1

Compositions of PBS and Ringer's solutions used in this study.

	PBS (g/L)	Ringer's (g/L)
NaCl	8.077	6.000
KCl	0.209	0.300
$NaH_2PO_4{}^*7H_2O$		
$CaCl_2{}^*2H2O$		0.200
$MgSO_4{}^*7H2O$		
$NaHCO_3$		
KH_2PO_4		
Glucose		
Na_2HPO_4	1.161	
KH_2PO_4	0.202	
$C_3H_5NaO_3$		3.100

Figure 1

Cyclic potentiodynamic polarization plots for Ti64+B alloys from OCP to 800mV in deaerated PBS measured at 37°C with reference to Ag/AgCl and recalculated with reference to SCE.

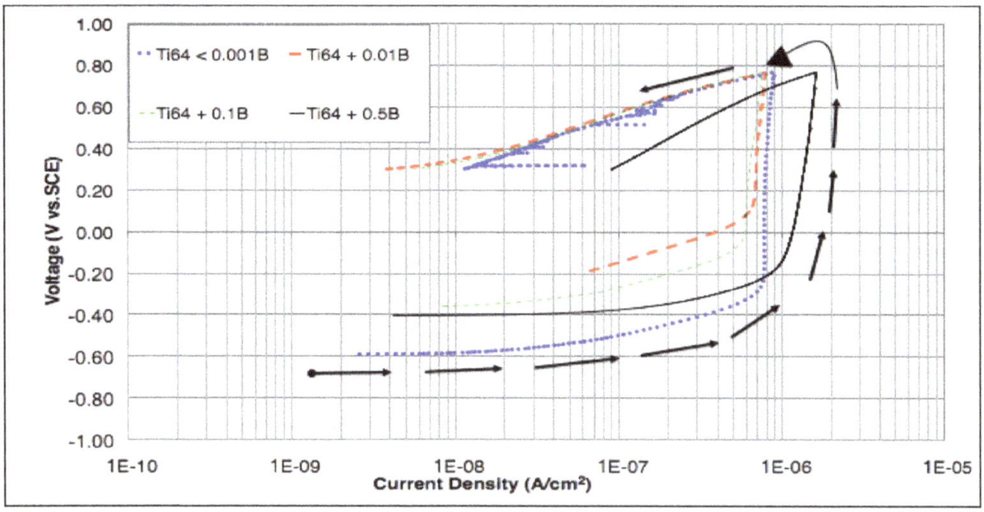

gas thirty minutes prior to testing and throughout the tests. The flow rate of nitrogen used during deaeration was reduced to accommodate for the smaller solution volume of 250 cm^3 as opposed to the 1000 cm^3 in the standard.

The F2129 tests were conducted using a commercially available potentiostat. The three-electrode flat cell was placed inside a copper Faraday cage to minimize electrical noise. The corrosion cell contained an Ag/AgCl reference electrode (+209 mV vs. SHE) with 3M NaCl as a filling solution, a platinum-coated niobium mesh counter electrode and the working electrode with an exposed surface area of 1 cm^2. All potential measurements were recorded with respect to the Ag/AgCl reference electrode. Subsequently, these values were recalculated with reference to the Saturated Calomel Electrode (SCE) [7], to be consistent with the standard.

The test began with a one hour Open Circuit Potential (OCP), followed by a Cyclic Potentiodynamic Polarization (CPP) scan in which the applied voltage was increased from the OCP to 800 mV and then decreased to the OCP again at a constant scan rate of 0.167 mV per second.

RESULTS AND DISCUSSION

Figures 1 - 3 show the results of the F2129 cyclic potentiodynamic polarization plots under deaerated, body temperature conditions from the OCP to 800 mV and a portion of the return scan to rest potential. The voltage readings in these figures were plotted relative to the saturated calomel electrode (SCE) (recalculated from data obtained with respect to the Ag/AgCl electrode). The plots were examined for signs of breakdown. All the OCP values were below zero, relative to SCE. This is consistent with another study regarding the electrochemical characterization of the same alloys, including CPTi, Ti64 and Ti67 in deaerated Ringer's solutions[12].

Figure 2

Cyclic potentiodynamic polarization plots for Ti64+B alloys from OCP to 800mV in deaerated Ringer's measured at 37°C with reference to Ag/AgCl in and recalculated with reference to SCE.

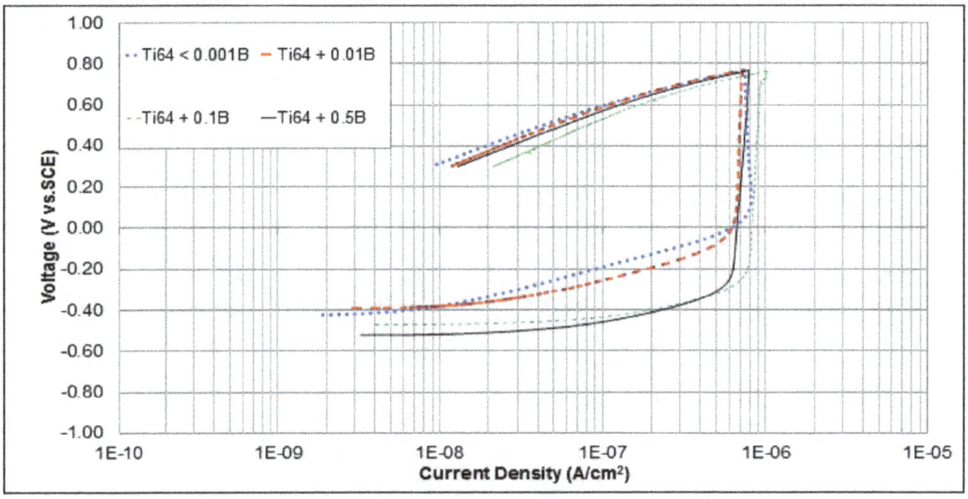

Figure 3

Cyclic potentiodynamic polarization plots for Ti64+B alloys from OCP to 800mV in deaerated DBS measured at 37°C with reference to Ag/AgCl and recalculated with reference to SCE.

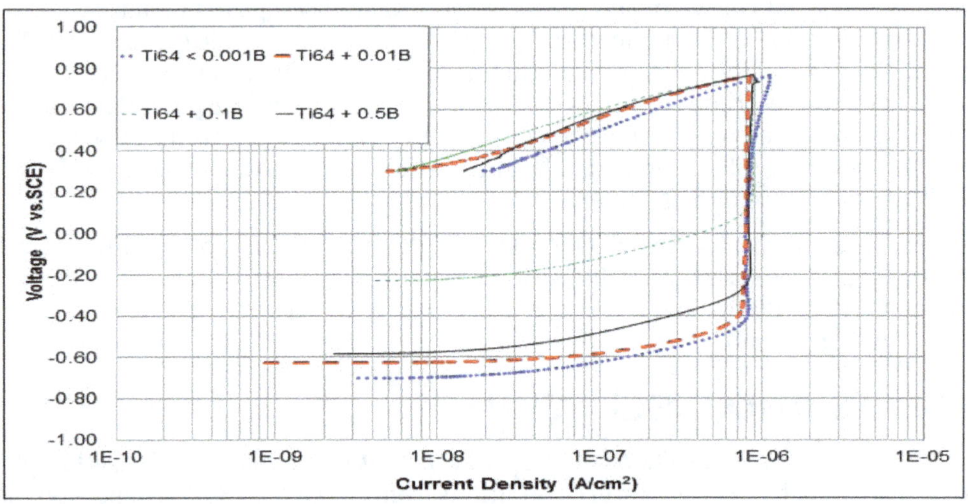

None of the Ti64+B alloys indicate any signs of the pitting, as evidenced by, (a) the near vertical forward curve at low (passive) current densities without evidence of breakdown (which would be seen as a dramatic increase in current density at the onset of pit initiation), and (b), the decline in current density upon reversal of polarization. Both (a) and (b) point to the formation of a protective oxide layer on the surface of these alloys. Therefore, all of the tested alloys passed the F2129 test and are potential candidates for biomedical implants.

Figure 4

E_{pass} measurement of Ti64 + B alloys in DBS solution.

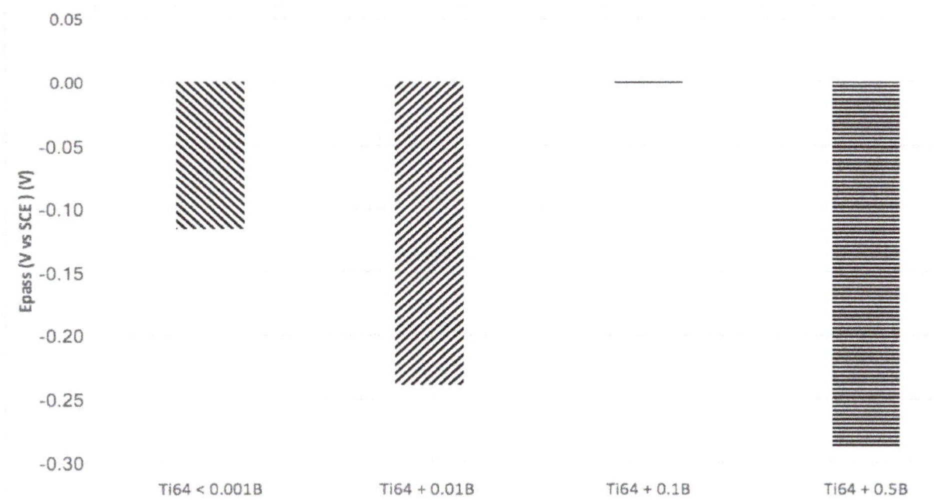

Figure 5

I_{pass} measurements of Ti64 + B alloys in DBS solution.

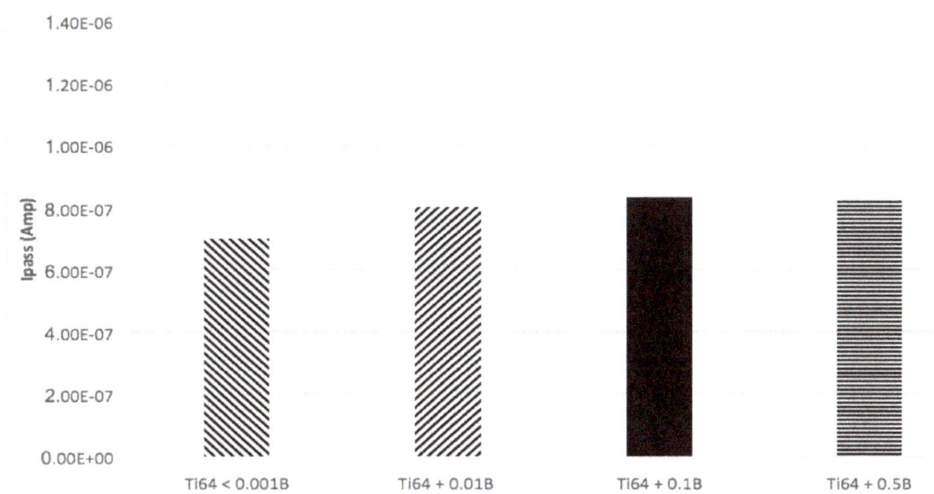

Examination of the post-tested coupons using an optical microscope showed no visible signs of pitting. Statistical analysis of the current at the passivation potential (I_{pass}) and the current at the vertex potential (I_{vertex}), showed that there wasn't a significant difference, at the 95% confidence level, between the I_{pass} and the I_{vertex} for most of these alloys. Therefore, the I_{pass} was considered to be constant. Notable exceptions were Ti64+0.1B and Ti64+0.5B in DBS.

Further insights into the corrosion behavior of these alloys can be attributed by extracting the value of the passivation potential (E_{pass}) and the corresponding current (I_{pass}). Examples in DBS and Ringer's solution are discussed below in Figures 4 - 7.

Figure 6

E_{pass} measurements of Ti64 + B alloys in Ringer's solution.

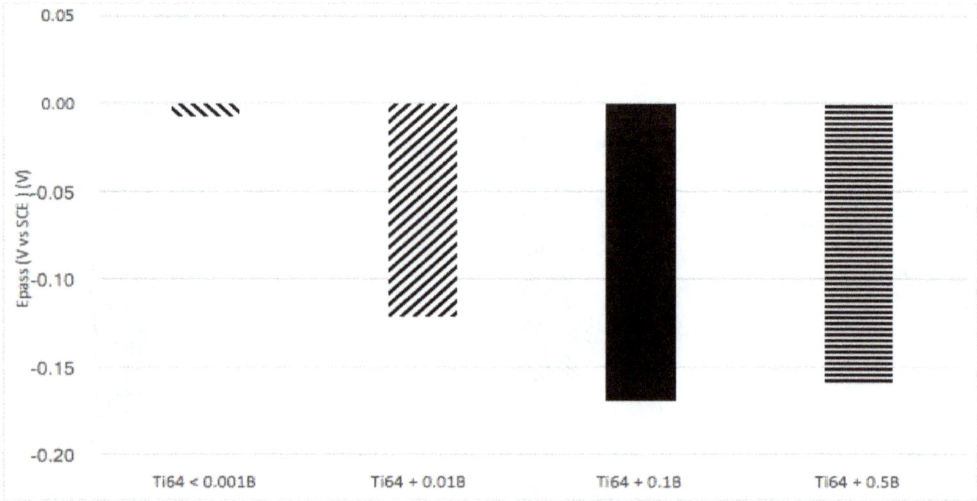

Figure 7

I_{pass} measurements of Ti64 + B alloys in Ringer's solution.

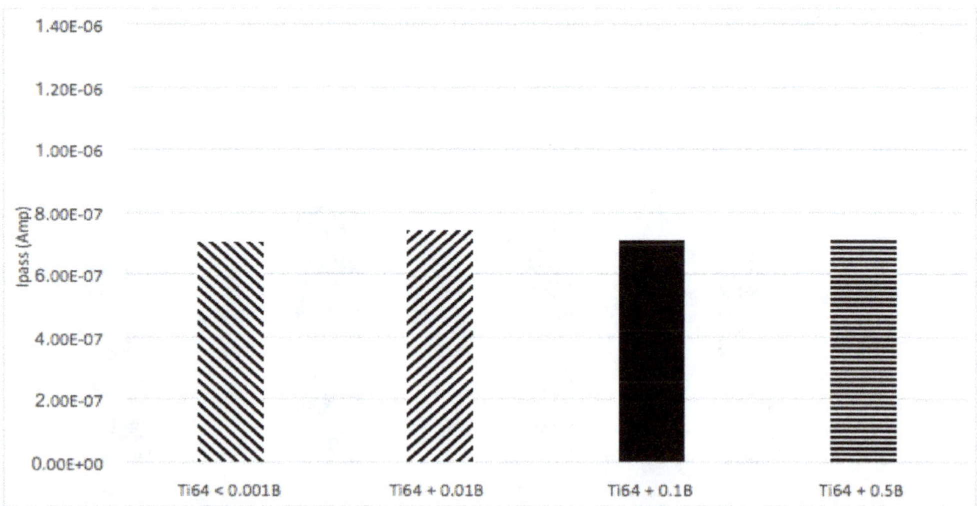

Figures 4 and 5 show the E_{pass} and I_{pass} of the Ti64 + B alloys in DBS solution. The E_{pass} decreased with increasing boron content, with the notable exception of Ti64 + 0.1B. The I_{pass} values show a slight increase with increasing boron content. Figure 6 and 7 shows the E_{pass} and I_{pass} of Ti64 + B alloys in Ringers solution. The E_{pass} also decreased with increasing boron amount, with the exception of Ti64 + 0.5B. I_{pass} values showed to have decreased for the higher boron amounts.

The major differences between PBS and Ringer's is the presence of sodium l-lactate and calcium chloride dihydrate in the latter and the disodium phosphate and potassium dihydrogen phosphates in the former. The exact composition of the DBS is not available; however, the solution constituents are quite different as noted in the experimental section. In addition, the starting pH of the PBS solution is nominally 7.31, the Ringer's is 6.36 and the DBS is 7.71. The pH at the end of the tests are 7.32, 6.34 and 8.31 for each of the solutions respectively. The pH differences are very small for the PBS (buffered) and the Ringer's (unbuffered) whereas the DBS became more basic. The compositional and pH differences could account for the differences in performance of the different alloys in these solutions.

CONCLUSIONS

Each of the alloys in this test matrix (Ti64, Ti64+0.01 wt% B, Ti64+0.1 wt% B and Ti64+0.05 wt% B) was subjected to a modified ASTM F2129-15 in three different solutions (PBS, DBS and Ringer's). The following key conclusions can be drawn from the above: (a) all alloys form and retain their passive layers across the tested potential range, and (b) small amounts of boron (0.01 wt% B) apparently decrease the minimum threshold voltage for passive layer formation in all solutions.

ACKNOWLEDGEMENTS

The authors would like to acknowledge Daniel Navarro, Grazziela Sena, Jacob Benoun, Jenny Wong, Adam Teoh, Joe Tulpinski and Ulus Ekerman (Cal Poly Pomona) and Jonathan Harris (Pomona College) for their support. We also want to acknowledge Cal Poly Pomona for their assistance during this project. The authors gratefully acknowledge financial support from Ms. Sylvia Hall, Drs. George and Mei Lai, the LA section of NACE International, Western States Corrosion Seminar, Western Area of NACE International, the NACE Foundation, California Steel Industries, Inc., and the Southern California Chapter of the Association for Iron & Steel Technology.

REFERENCES

1. Rack H.J. and Qazi J.I., "Titanium alloys for biomedical applications," *Materials Science and Engineering:* C 26, 8 (2006): p. 1269.
2. Gallo J., et al., "Recent Advances in Arthroplasty: Aseptic Loosening of Total Hip Arthroplasty as a Result of Local Failure of Tissue Homeostasis," in *Recent Advances in Arthroplasty*, ed. Fokter Samo K. (Rijeka, Croatia: Intech, 2012) pp. 319-354.
3. Mohammed M.T., Khan Z.A., Siddiquee A.N., "Beta Titanium Alloys: The Lowest Elastic Modulus for Biomedical Applications: A Review," *International Journal of Chemical, Molecular, Nuclear, Materials and Metallurgical Engineering* 8, 8 (2014): pp. 781-786.
4. Nielsen F. H., "Update on human health effects of boron" *Journal of Trace Elements in Medicine and Biology* 28, 4 (2014): pp. 383-387.
5. Mastromatteo E., Sullivan F., "Summary: International Symposium on the Health Effects of Boron and Its Compounds." *Environmental Health Perspectives* (1994): pp. 139-141.
6. Ravi V.A., Rogers S., Malek M., Surmenian D., Priddy I., Harrison B., Schissler A., Divi S.C., Tamirisakandala S., Miracle D., "The Environmental Stability of Boron-Containing Titanium Alloys for Biomedical Applications." *Journal of Materials* 63, 6 (2011): p. 42-47.

7. Ravi V.A., Wantah W., Castenada S., Permana B., Rey G., Alas S., Morin K., Tamirisa S., Miracle D., "Corrosion and Immune Response Of Boron-Modified Titanium Alloys In Biological Environments." Corrosion/2009, paper no. 09466 (Houston, TX: NACE, 2009), pp. 1-16.
8. Ravi V.A., Schissler A., Chantrjaroen W., Beecher C., Razzak A., Urak R., Alas S., "Corrosion Behavior and Biocompatibility of Boron Containing Titanium Alloys in Simulated Physiological Environments." *Corrosion Engineering, Science, and Technology* 47, 5 (2012): pp. 383-387.
9. McCann K., Miguel J., Margoosian G., Voorhees T., Ravi V., "Electrochemical Evaluation of Titanium-Boron Alloys for Potential Biomedical Applications," Corrosion/2016, paper no. 7842, (Houston, TX: NACE, 2016), pp. 1-12.
10. Voorhees T., Villalpando O., Ravi V. A., "Characterization of the Corrosion Behavior of Advanced Titanium Alloys in Simulated Physiological Environments Using Electrochemical Impedance Spectroscopy," Corrosion/2015, paper no. 6120 (Houston, Texas: NACE, 2015), pp. 1-10.
11. ASTM F2129-15. "*Standard Test Method for Conducting Cyclic Potentiodynamic Polarization Measurements to Determine the Corrosion Susceptibility of Small Implant Devices.*" (West Conshohocken, PA: ASTM, 2015), pp. 1-9.
12. Cai Z., Shafer T., Watanabe I., Nunn M. E., Okabe T., "Electrochemical Characterization of Cast Titanium Alloys," *Biomaterials* 24, 2 (2003): pp. 213-218.

Paper Number:
C2017-09584

Graphene Based Nanomaterials for Biomedical Coatings

Rigoberto C. Advincula

Department of Macromolecular Science and Engineering

Abstract

Nanotechnology involves scale, function, and composition that enable macroscopic properties with improved performance and high-value adding for any industry including the biomedical industry. The use of graphene-based nanomaterials is of high interest for electronic applications and the solid-state display industry. However, it is not as well known in the biomedical and bio-implant field. The graphene and the oxidized graphene oxide GO nanomaterials can be prepared by plasma, vacuum deposition, solid state catalytic methods, and also by solution exfoliation methods. This paper highlights work done on utilizing GO coatings and dispersions as anti-microbial and protective barriers for preventing biocorrosion and biofilm growth. Utilizing surface analytical tools including electrochemical methods it is possible to characterize their ultrathin properties based on electro-deposited and LB deposited films. They have been shown to have good anti-microbial properties against gram + and gram - bacteria and have been benign against fibroblast mammalian cells.

Keywords: graphene, coatings, anti-microbial, anti-corrosion

INTRODUCTION

Since the awarding of the Physics Nobel Prize in 2010, graphene, a two-dimensional carbon polymorph nanomaterial has continued to be the subject of much intense research. There has been interest worldwide for both fundamental properties and applications. Other carbon based polymorphs such as carbon nanotubes (CNT)s and fullerene – another Nobel Prize winning discovery followed much earlier are much more commercially available. Elemental Carbon (C) naturally comes in two basic allotropes, namely graphite and diamond. These are two very different materials based on their chemical orbital hybridization and crystallinity despite being all carbon atoms. But as nanomaterials, they exhibit extraordinary electronic properties and are of primary interest to the materials community. There is a lot of interest now in utilizing them for future flexible electronic displays and devices.

Graphene a, 2D nanomaterial has unusual electrical and optical properties (Figure 1). It is a single layer of carbon atoms arranged in an aromatic hexagonal lattice resulting in high mobilities and charge carrier generation. This arises of course from the delocalization and hybridization of pi-orbitals in a vast planar network of fused benzene like structures. It is an ideal monolayer coating material due to its impermeability, thermodynamic stability, transparency and flexibility. They exhibit high field effect mobility and can be formed through a number of chemical and physical methods and can be rendered useful in batch compounding. Its potential applications have encompassed a myriad of scientific and engineering disciplines such as high-performance nanocomposites, printed and flexible electronics, supercapacitors, chemical sensors, gas barriers and biomaterials. The latter include applications in gene and drug delivery, cancer treatment, cell growth control, stem cell differentiation, field effect transistor (FET) -based biosensors and as antimicrobial materials.

Figure 1

Differentiation of the heavily pi-electron delocalized 2D nanomaterial (G) and the highly oxidized but functionality rich graphene oxide (GO).

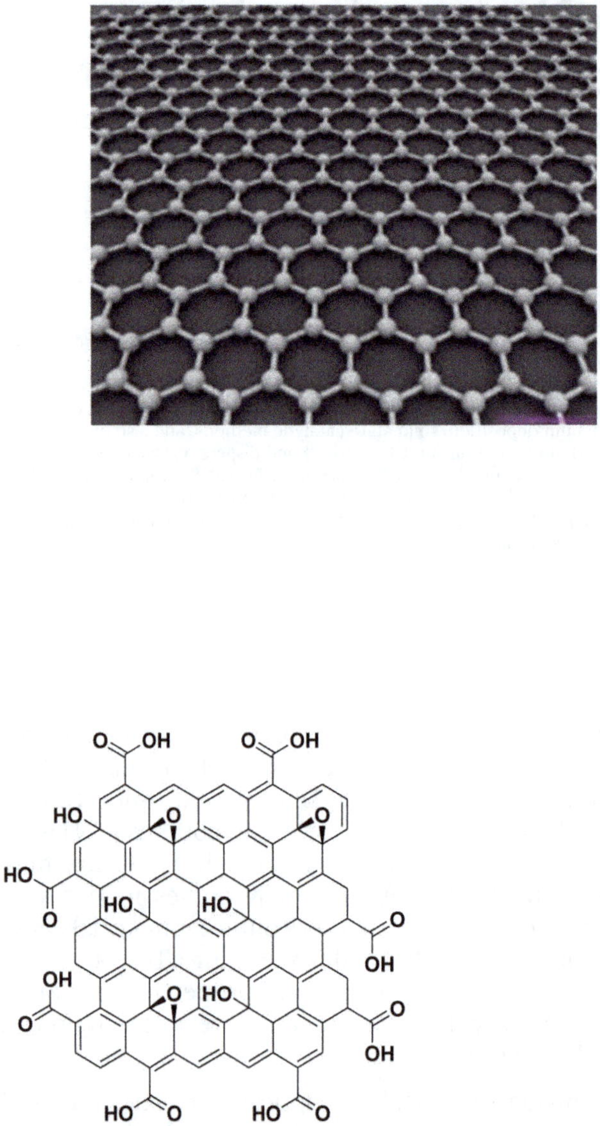

Specifically of high interest to corrosion technologists is the use of graphene as barrier materials for preventing corrosion or even biocorrosion. Atomically thin layers of graphene can serve as a protective coating that inhibits corrosion of underlying metals. Electrochemical methods can be employed to study the corrosion inhibition on steel, copper and nickel by either growing graphene on these metals directly (plasma or chemical vapor deposition) or by mechanically transferring multilayer graphene onto them based on solution or dispersion chemistry. Cyclic voltammetry (CV) measurements, electrochemical impedance spectroscopy (EIS) measurements, and Tafel analysis can be used to determine the mechanism and quantify the corrosion rates of graphene based coatings. It can yet be thinnest known corrosion-protecting coating that is commercially viable.

For biomedical devices and therapeutic patch applications, coating materials with anti-bacterial properties are of high interest. In several studies, we have shown that graphene and its derivatives exhibit antimicrobial potency as dispersions or coatings. Particularly, graphene oxide (GO) (Figure 1), a heavily oxidized derivative of graphene, contains various oxygen-rich functionalities that impart excellent solution processability and sites for further chemical modification, thereby facilitating its applications in many areas especially in biomedicine. These functional groups include epoxide, hydroxyl, carboxylic functionality, and partially saturated C-C linkages. Our group has reported a number of reports on the cytotoxicity and antimicrobial effect of graphene, GO nanocomposites and their derivatives. [2-5] Decorating nanoparticles on any surface with GO further improves its antimicrobial effect. The mechanism by which pure graphene and graphene oxide act as antimicrobial agents is of high interest and may go through several routes. This may go through the generation of RO radical species, basal plane or edge effects of the nanomaterial against colonization, breaking or contribution to the REDOX cycle and ion transport on membrane protein-channels on the membrane surface.

EXPERIMENTAL

Characterization Methods: This paper does not detail the specific experimental tools and the experiments that produced the results. Rather the list is made of the instrumentation used in a number of studies. For detailed instrumentation and methodologies with the specific topics, please refer to the original papers. [1-5] A number of surface analytical microscopic and spectroscopic methods were applied to enable full characterization of films and coatings prior to any corrosion or anti-microbial studies. Characterization includes: UV-vis spectroscopy for absorbance measurements (correlated conversion from graphene (G) to graphene oxide (GO), Scanning Electron Microscopy (SEM) and Atomic Force Microscopy (AFM) analysis for morphology of GO and direct bacterial imaging, static water contact angle for wetting (determine surface energy of film), FT-IR spectroscopy measurements as well as IR-imaging for chemical functional group determination (verify conversion of G to GO). X-ray photoelectron spectroscopy (XPS) for surface elemental analysis (characterization of film), and thermogravimetric analysis (TGA) for determination of relative compositions and weight degradation of GO preparation. AFM measurements in particular were conducted using a PicoScan 2500 AFM (Agilent Technologies) with a piezo scanner or a Park AFM NX-10 system under tapping (non-contact) mode

Synthesis of GO. Again, a general procedure is described here and further specifics on the procedure can be found in our original papers. The synthesis of GO was performed based on the well-known Hummers Method. Graphite flakes in concentrated H_2SO_4 were allowed to mix in a round-bottom flask (RBF) for 10 min. Then, $KMnO_4$ was slowly added to the reaction mixture, which immediately turned dark green upon addition of $KMnO_4$ after every 24 h of mixing. The reaction was stopped and the reaction mixture was mixed in ice-water mixture. After which, H_2O_2 was slowly added, which turned the dark purple solution to yellow. The solution was placed in centrifuge tubes and was then centrifuged for separation. The supernate was discarded, and the sediments were washed with purified water once followed by centrifugation. Further purification steps were performed using isopropanol.

DATA AND RESULTS

There have been several methods reported to prepare ultrathin film coatings made up G, GO and reduced graphene oxide (rGO) compositions. A number of these methods are specific for making very thin to monolayers with large monodomain sizes or relative thick films. The films can be evaluated for their thickness, refractive index and optical properties, surface morphology, and homogeneity prior to any corrosion or anti-microbial property studies. This includes: 1) Spin casting of a dispersion of the nanomaterials in a particular solvent, 2) multicomponent formulation of the GO with an existing polymer or emulsion that can result in high and relatively thick film forming properties, 3) Vacuum or plasma synthesis using a catalyst and a carbon source at high temperature or pressures, 4) Direct carbonization with high temperature or combustion as thin films, and 5) by Langmuir-Blodgett (LB) deposition methods at the air-water interface. 6) formation of layer-by-layer ultrathin films of GO with polyelectrolytes. Deposition studies have been done on flat substrate surfaces: glass, Si-wafer, titanium alloys, silicones, and treated poly(ethylene terephthalate) (PET) substrates.

In general for our experiments, the GO can be synthesized by chemical exfoliation of graphite using the classic modified Hummers and Offeman's method. The final product can be characterized by UV-Vis, Raman Spectroscopy, IR, and XPS. AFM and SEM can be used to confirm the orientation of GO with respect to the substrate.

In one study, we demonstrated a blend composition of polyvinylcarbazole-graphene (PVK-G) solutions to form ultrathin films and their unique anti-microbial properties (Figure 2).[1,2] Highly dispersed PVK-G (97/3 w/w %) homogeneous solutions in various organic and aqueous solvents were prepared by solution mixing and sonication methods. FTIR and X-ray diffraction (XRD) were used to characterize the presence of GO functional groups and the formation of the nanocomposite polymers. These films demonstrated excellent bacterial toxicity with low cytotoxicity to human cells. They should be strong candidates for biomaterials applications. The thermal properties and morphology of the nanocomposites were analyzed using TGA and AFM, respectively. PVK-G films were electrodeposited and electropolymerized onto indium tin oxide (ITO) substrates via. Cyclic voltammetry (CV) and UV-Vis were used to monitor the electrodeposition process. AFM was used to characterize the morphology of the nanocomposite thin film that was deposited on ITO.

Antimicrobial property of the electrodeposited PVK-G films and solution-based PVK-G were investigated against *Escherichia coli (E. coli) and Bacillus subtillis (B. subtillis)*. The PVK-G was investigated for: 1) quantitative microbial growth after exposure to the nanocomposite, 2) metabolic assay, and 3) live-dead assay of the bacterial solutions. In all cases, PVK-G material presented fewer viable and active bacteria than those exposed to PVK and graphene solution controls (Figure 3). Biofilm growth and colonization was monitored (perhaps a mechanism against quorum sensing). The PVK-G film inhibited about eighty percent of biofilm surface coverage while the PVK and G-modified surfaces separately allowed biofilm formation in almost the whole coated surface (i.e. >80 %) as observed by AFM (Figure 4). The biocompatibility or cytotoxicity of the

Figure 2

Preparation of exfoliated PVK-G dispersions and thin films and their anti-microbial properties. Figure from reference [8].

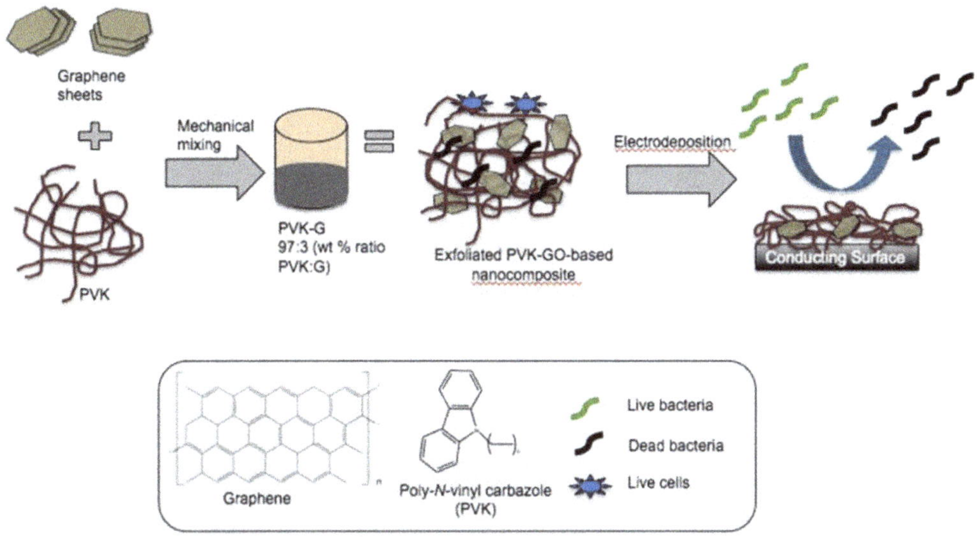

Figure 3

(a) The cytotoxic effect of nanomaterials against NIH-3T3 Fibroblast cells was investigated by an MTS assay method. The results after twenty-four hours exposure of the fibroblast cells to PVK-G and PVK solutions are shown. (b) The toxicity effect of PVK-G (97/3 w/w % and at various concentrations with PVK and graphene solutions on *E. coli and B. subtilis.* Figures from Ref. [8]

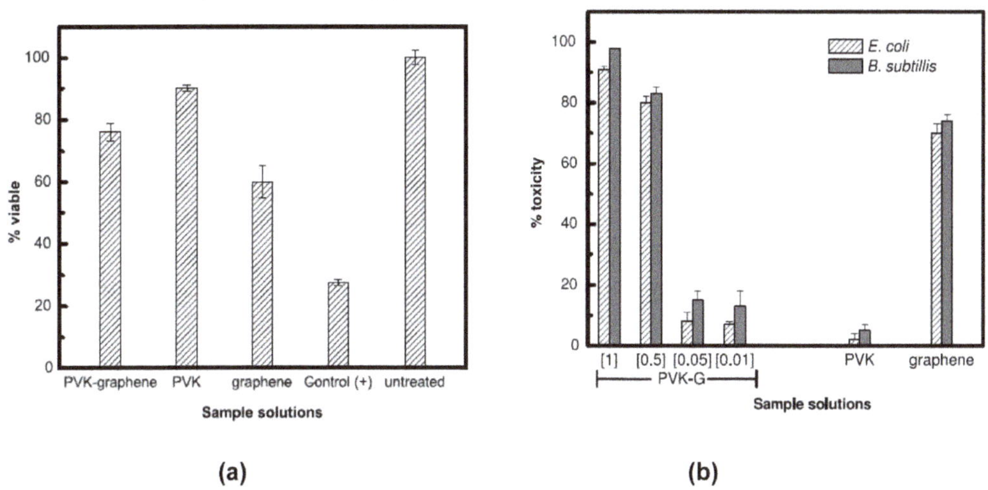

prepared PVK-G solutions on NIH 3T3 cells was evaluated using the MTS assay method. The 24 h exposure of the PVK-G nanocomposite to the NIH-3T3 cells presented about eighty percent cell survival indicating less toxicity or high survivability (Figure 3). [1,2]

In another study, the objective was to determine whether the edges or basal plane of GO play an important role in its antimicrobial mechanism [6]. The LB technique was used to deposit planarized graphene oxide (GO) sheets on a PET substrate. The

Figure 4

Biofilm formation studies on surface coated with PVK-G film. AFM topography (top) and friction images (bottom) of (a) PVK-G, (b) PVK, and (c) bare ITO surfaces after 24 h incubation with E. coli. Scale bar: 20 micron. Figure from Ref. [7].

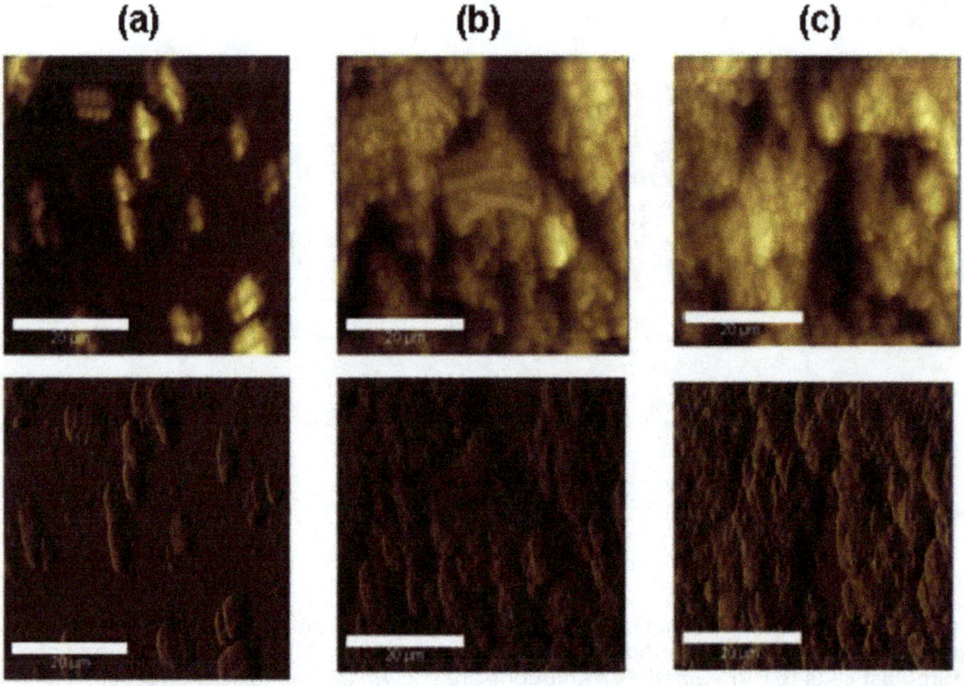

results of the study suggested that the antibacterial activity is not necessarily derived from the contact with the edges of the GO but from the exposure to the basal planes of the nanomaterials. Controlling the number of layers or the orientation of the GO nanomaterials can increase the pathogenic toxicity response. These findings highlighted the importance of the basal plane in the bacterial death mechanism.[6]

To demonstrate the use of GO in heavy metal cleanup simultaneous with anti-microbial properties, we have reported the synthesis and evaluation of a number of graphene oxide thin films and their antimicrobial properties.[7] The goal is to demonstrate the possibility for other types of filtration and purification applications with anti-microbial properties. In this study, a specific derivative of GO, GO-EDTA was synthesized for chelating and capture of heavy metals and dispersions and thin films prepared. The antimicrobial activity of graphene oxide silanized with N-(trimethoxysilylpropyl) ethylenediamine triacetic acid (GO–EDTA) against Gram-negative, *Cupriavidus metallidurans* CH4, and Gram-positive bacteria, *Bacillus subtilis*, was demonstrated. Cytotoxicity to human corneal epithelial cell line *hTCEpi* was also tested. The results showed that GO–EDTA improved anti-microbial properties when compared to graphene oxide (GO) alone. About 92.3 ± 10% and 99.1 ± 1.3% cell inactivation of *B. subtilis* and *C. metallidurans* was observed respectively. The mechanism for bacterial inactivation was attributed to cell oxidative stress mechanisms. No cytotoxicity was observed towards human corneal epithelial cell lines hTCEp after 24 h exposure to GO–EDTA. This means that these materials have potential for applications that can involve human exposure and are relatively harmless.

To demonstrate pollution and heavy metal cleanup, GO- EDTA's adsorption capacity for two heavy metals, Cu2+ and Pb2+ at different concentrations, pH, and contact time were investigated. The maximum adsorption capacity of the GO–EDTA was determined to be 454.6 mg g^{-1} and 108.7 mg g^{-1} for Pb^{2+} and Cu^{2+}, respectively, exceeding the capacity of traditional adsorbent materials, such as activated carbon.

Lastly, we have reported the room temperature fabrication of graphene nanomesh (GNM) via a colloidal templating approach. This offered a facile and accurate control of array formation by simply varying the size of the colloidal template. The colloidal particles were prepared using an LB like deposition method to form a hexagonally-closed pack array or pattern. Traditionally, electrochemical oxidative etching (EOE) was employed to puncture holes on the graphene sheet. By demonstrating this concept, one can prepare various patterned films, which can change their semi-conductor behavior and porosity as films. [4]

CONCLUSIONS

We have reported a number of approaches to prepare nanomaterials and thin film nanocomposites of G, GO, and rGO derivatives. They can be prepared as spin-casted films, electropolymerized thin films, patterned thin films, and Langmuir-Blodgette deposited films. More importantly, we have demonstrated their anti-microbial properties and ability to prevent the formation of biofilms. Their current behavior against anti-corrosion properties is being evaluated by our laboratory and will be reported soon. We intend to demonstrate possible applications of various nanocomposite formulations in 3-D printed parts that may find utility as materials and coatings for tissue scaffolding and bio-implant design.

ACKNOWLEDGEMENTS

This work was made possible by the hard work of the Advincula Research Group members in particular Dr. Joey Mangadlao who developed projects on the synthesis and testing of graphene based dispersions and developed a number of analytical methodologies in the laboratory. We also thank Prof. Debora Rodrigues for our long-standing collaboration with her group on most of the bio-assay studies. Technical support from Park AFM Systems, Malvern Instruments, Biolin Scientific, Agilent Technologies (now Keysight Technologies) and Thales Nano are greatly acknowledged.

REFERENCES

1. Santos C., Vergara C. A., Cui K., Pernites R., Advincula R., "Fabrication and characterization of electrodeposited thin films from highly dispersed poly(N-vinylcarbazole) (PVK)-graphene oxide (GO) nanocomposites" *Macromol. Chem. Phys.*, 212, (2011): p. 2371.
2. Santos C., Tria C., Vergara A., Ahmed F., Advincula R., Rodrigues D.D., "Antimicrobial graphene polymer (PVK-GO) nanocomposite films" *Chem. Comm.*, 47, (2011):p. 8892-8894.
3. Mangadlao J., de Leon A., Felipe M., Cao P., Advincula P., Advincula R., "Grafted Carbazole-Assisted Electrodeposition of Graphene Oxide." ACS *Appl. Mater. Interfaces*, 7 (2015): p. 10266.
4. Mangadlao J., de Leon A., Felipe M., Advincula R., "Electrochemical fabrication of graphene nanomesh via colloidal templating." *Chem. Commun.*, 51, (2015): p. 7629.

5. Santos C., Mangadlao J., Ahmed F., Leon A., Advincula R., Rodrigues D., "Graphene nanocomposite for biomedical applications: fabrication, antimicrobial and cytotoxic investigations" *Nanotechnology*, 23, (2012): p. 395101.
6. Mangadlao J., Santos C., Felipe J., Leon A., Rodrigues R., Advincula R. D., "On the Antibacterial Mechanism of Graphene Oxide Langmuir Blodgett Films" *Chemical Communications*, 51, (2015): p. 2886.
7. Carpio I., Mangadlao J., Nguyen H., Advincula R., Rodrigues D.D., "Graphene oxide functionalized with ethylenediamine triacetic acid for heavy metal adsorption and anti-microbial applications". *Carbon*, 77, (2014): p. 289.
8. Santos C., Mangadlao J., Ahmed F., Leon A., Advincula R., Rodrigues D., "Graphene nanocomposite for biomedical applications: fabrication, antimicrobial and cytotoxic investigations" *Nanotechnology*, 23, (2012): p. 395101.

Paper Number:
C2021-16540

Electrochemical Testing of Additive Manufactured Ti6Al4V and NiTi Materials in a Biological Fluid Environment

Elizabeth Trillo
Southwest Research Institute

Carl Popelar
Southwest Research Institute

Abstract

The use of additive manufacturing (AM) has seen a marked increase in the biomedical arena for hip and knee replacements, especially for older populations. The AM method is particularly attractive in the biomedical industry as it allows for patient specific designs in the case of unusual anatomy. AM also is well suited to manufacture highly complex parts and has the benefit of rapid prototyping and rapid manufacturing. However, as the increase in fabrication and use of these components have increased, there are still some underlying corrosion issues that have yet to be fully understood. This research looks at the electrochemical polarization behavior of AM fabricated UNS R56401 (Ti6Al4V) and NiTi (Nitinol) in a biological fluid. Different build orientations were evaluated as well as different post processing and different surface roughness. Cyclic polarization testing was performed per ASTM F2129[1] in a Phosphate Buffered Saline solution at 99 F. Surface roughness evaluations were performed prior to testing as well as Scanning Electron Microscopy (SEM) prior to and after testing.

Keywords: Additive Manufacturing, Ti6Al4V, NiTi, Electrochemical Testing, Biomedical

INTRODUCTION

Additive Manufacturing (AM), also known as 3-D printing, is a process by which a component is fabricated layer by layer.[2,3] It boasts many benefits over conventional processing (casting) methods such as being able to fabricate complex components, flexibility to create drastically different components in the same build space, rapid prototyping, rapid manufacturing and ability to change the design without costly changes to the processing chain. The lure of these benefits has affected major industries such as aerospace, automotive, biomedical and to an increasing extent oil and gas industry, with the goal of producing final products from the AM machine in each of these sectors.

UNS R56401 (Ti6Al4V) is often used as an orthopedic material for hip replacements, femoral, knee joint constructions as well as for dental and mandible implants.[4-10] It is suitable as a biomaterial due to its high strength-to-weight ratio, high corrosion resistance, and biocompatibility.[11] Conventional manufacturing of these products are in standard sizes, which may not be optimally suited for each individual body. Improper sizing can lead to uneven stress distribution of the implant to the load bearing bone as well as contributing to micro-motion of the implant that would lead to lack of biocompatibility (cell adhesion and proliferation). At the same time, the goal of the final implantation is to maximize contact between bone and implant to ensure multiple points for cell adhesion. Thus, additive manufacturing of Ti6Al4V implants seem like an attractive processing step for successful implantation as it would allow to design and build for a specific patient anatomy.

Figure 1

Diagram showing the Ti6Al4V AM coupon build. Arrow represents the direction of the coater.

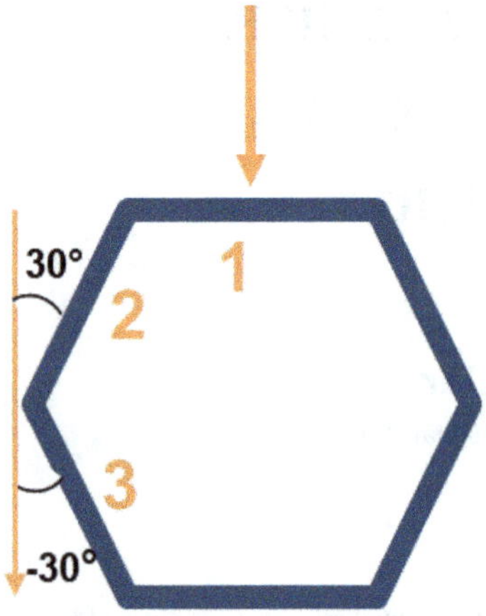

Corrosion studies of AM fabricated Ti6Al4V have centered around differences in selective laser melting (SLM) and electron beam melting (EBM) methods[12,13], or looked at fine polishing only[14], whereas others have looked at Ti6Al4V but in different types of environments.[15] For Nitinol, limited research has been performed, and has focused on the effects of a polished (not as-fabricated) surface.[16] But these efforts have not considered other factors that can affect the corrosion behavior of an AM build. One such factor is the orientation of an AM build. Although work is emerging on the impacts of sample orientation and location of the part on the build plate, a consideration must be given to the resulting surface structure and how it impacts the corrosion capabilities. Other factors such as powder size, AM build process parameters (laser power, and scan velocity), along with post processing steps of the AM products (such as stress relieving, HIP and surface finish) can lead to differences in material microstructure and surface characteristics.

This research will compare the corrosion behavior of Ti6Al4V AM samples oriented at different angles on the build plate. Comparisons were made between the as-fabricated samples to polished samples and also to wrought Ti6Al4V ELI sample as a baseline. The corrosion behavior of NiTi (Nitinol) samples in the three different orientations were also evaluated. Cyclic polarization testing was performed with optical and scanning electron microscopy (SEM) on the sample surfaces after exposure to identify surface corrosion characteristics.

EXPERIMENTAL PROCEDURE

A hollow hexagon shaped sample made of Ti6Al4V ELI (UNS R56401) powder was fabricated using a Renishaw AM250 Selective Laser Melting (SLM) Powder Bed Fusion machine. The Ti6Al4V powder size was -16 /+45µm. The sides of the hexagon represented different orientations on the build plate, with 1 C orientation being perpendicular to the coater, 2 C 30° from the coater and 3 C a -30° from the coater (Figure 1).

The Nitinol AM sample was fabricated from -20/+60 µm powder. A cube sample was fabricated such that the different build surface faces could be tested. The X, Y, and Z surfaces were tested, with the Z axis representing the build direction as seen in Figure 2.

Figure 2

Diagram showing the Nitinol AM coupon build. Samples tested in the three different orientations.

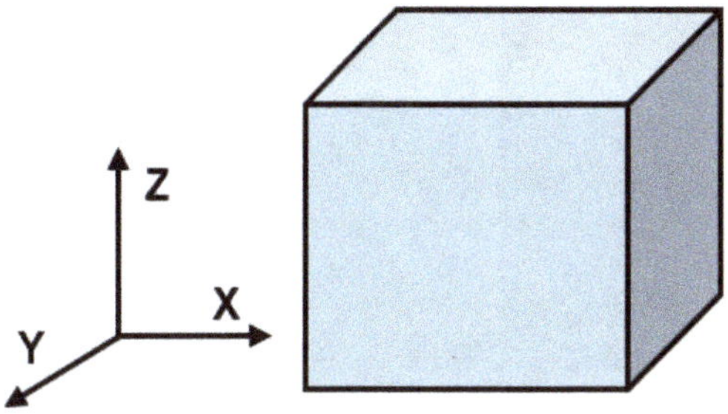

The surface roughness was performed both on the as-fabricated and polished sides using a Keyence VR 3000 G2 machine. In addition, the surface structure of the samples was observed via SEM after cyclic polarization (CP) testing.

Cyclic Potentiodynamic Polarization Testing was performed per ASTM F2129[1]. The test solution was phosphate buffered saline (pH 7.4) previously deaerated overnight with Nitrogen. Testing was conducted at 37°C (99 F) under a flow of Nitrogen gas. An Ag/AgCl electrode was used as the reference electrode while a Pt mesh acted as the counter electrode. The scan rate was 0.167 mV/sec. Since this was preliminary testing, only one scan rate was selected. After a minimum of one hour at the open circuit potential (E_{oc}), the sample went through a forward scan and reversed at 2.5V until the E_{oc} was reached. For the Ti6Al4V samples, duplicate measurements were performed on the as-fabricated outer diameter (Outside or OD) side while a single scan was performed on the inner diameter (ID) side of the sample that was polished to a 1200 grit finish. A wrought Ti6Al4V sample that was also polished to 1200 grit was utilized for comparison. Polarization scans were also performed on all three NiTi directions (X, Y, and Z) in the as-fabricated and polished conditions.

RESULTS

Ti6Al4V

The results of the surface roughness (Ra) measurements are presented in Table 1 for the Ti6Al4V samples. The Ra values were very similar for the as-fabricated samples oriented differently to the coater (90°, 30°, and -30°) with values ranging from 7 to 14 µm. It should also be noted that the as-fabricated OD and ID sides also had very similar surface roughness values. The polished samples, on the other hand, all had Ra values less than 1 µm, which in most cases was more than an order of magnitude lower than the as-fabricated samples.

Figure 3 shows the SEM micrographs of the surface morphology of the three different Ti6Al4V orientations in the as-fabricated state. The samples displayed typical surface condition of an AM sample prepared by powder bed fusion in that powders are partially melted on to the sample surface, along with river patters indicative of the melt by SLM.

Cyclic polarization testing on the Ti6Al4V AM samples in the as-fabricated state showed open circuit potentials (E_{oc}) in the range of -0.178 V to 0.144 V (as seen in Table 2 and Figure 4). The pitting potential (E_{pit}) was very similar for all as-fabricated samples with potentials between 2.09 V to 2.31 V. Pitting was verified visually after

Figure 3

SEM photographs showing surface structure of as-fabricated Ti6Al4V samples prior to testing in the a) 1C (90°), b) 2C (30°) and c) 3C (-30°) directions at 500x.

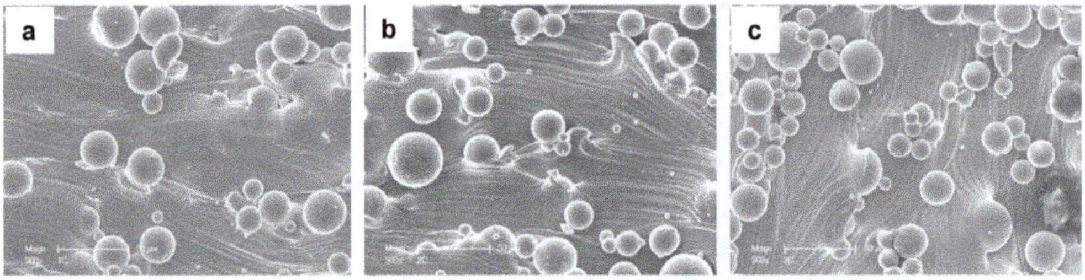

exposure (Figure 4b). The repassivation potential (E_{rp}) was approximately 1.5 V for all sample orientations. There was some variation in the passive currents of the samples. In addition, most samples also displayed a disruption in the passive region in the curve, indicating only pseudo-passive behavior (Figure 4a). The polished AM samples seen in Figure 5a, had much lower passive currents and were much more stable (i.e., no passive disruption) than the as-fabricated state. The pitting potential was only reached by one of the samples prior to the reverse scan indicating that the polished samples would have a higher pitting potential. Similarly, the wrought Ti6Al4V sample had the same low passive currents as the polished AM samples. The pitting potential was not reached on these samples as well before the reverse scan, also indicating higher pitting potentials than the as-fabricated Ti6Al4V (Figure 5).

SEM was performed on the as-fabricated samples after cyclic polarization testing in order to determine if there was a feature on the fracture surface that would account for the disturbances in the passive portion of the curves. In areas around the pit, there were instances of crevice corrosion that occurred in the crevice between the partially melted powder and the bulk surface, as well as near overlap areas of the melt (Figures 6

Table 1

Surface Roughness Measurements for Ti6Al4V Samples.

Material / Orientation	Surface Condition	Avg Ra, µm	Avg Rp, µm	Avg Rv, µm
Ti6Al4V – 1C (90°)	As Fabricated – OD	10	57	27
	As Fabricated – ID	13	71	39
	Polished – ID	0.90		
Ti6Al4V – 2C (30°)	As Fabricated – OD	7	47	22
	As Fabricated – ID	7	39	24
	Polished – ID	0.97		
Ti6Al4V – 3C (-30°)	As Fabricated – OD	9	44	35
	As Fabricated – ID	14	79	28
	Polished – ID	0.79		
Ti6Al4V – Wrought	Polished	0.68		

through 8). Light salt deposits were sometimes observed in these areas as well. In one case, it was observed that the partially melted powder sphere itself was preferentially corroding (Figure 8b).

Nitinol

The surface roughness for the Nitinol sample is seen in Table 3. The Ra values of as-fabricated were between 15 µm and 21 µm on the three different build orientations, which did not show great differences. The largest change was, of course, when the samples were polished. The Ra values were reduced by more than an order of magnitude, similar to Ti6Al4V. The as-fabricated surface morphology was also similar showing partial melting of powder on the sample surface as seen in the SEM photographs in Figure 9. The Z direction also showed evidence of the laser trail at lower magnification.

The cyclic polarization testing for the NiTi AM samples in the as-fabricated and polished state are seen in Figure 10. The E_{oc} values were between -0.022 V and 0.084 V for the as-fabricated samples and -0.136 V and -0.084 V (Table 4) for the polished samples. The forward scan showed passive behavior for the polished samples and a pseudo passive behavior for the as-fabricated samples. Both the polished and as-fabricated then showed a marked increase in current density, followed by a lower slope increase at higher current densities. The reverse scan showed repassivation potentials (E_{rp}) that were very close for the as-fabricated samples (1.01 V to 1.09 V) and was 0.956 V to 0.986 V for the polished samples. There was thus little change in these parameters for the three different sample orientations. The passive currents were somewhat higher for the X and Y orientations compared to the Z orientation for the as fabricated condition. The X and Y orientations also displayed disruptions in the passive curve, while the Z direction and the polished samples did not. The polished samples all displayed the same passive region which was similar to the lower value

Table 2

Cyclic Polarization Data for Ti6Al4V Samples.

Sample Identification	Surface Condition	Eocp, V	Epit, V	Erp, V
1C2 - 90°	As-Fabricated Outside A	-0.178	2.31	1.58
2C2 - 30°	As-Fabricated Outside A	-0.100	2.25	1.56
2C2 - 30°	As-Fabricated Outside B	-0.019	2.09	1.53*
3C2 - -30°	As-Fabricated Outside A	-0.155	2.28	1.52
3C2 - -30°	As-Fabricated Outside B	0.144	2.25	1.54
1C2 - 90°	Polished – ID	-0.062	--	--
2C2 - 30°	Polished – ID	-0.153	2.48	--
3C2 - -30°	Polished – ID	-0.035	--	--
Wrought	Polished – A	0,040	--	--
Wrought	Polished – B	-0.025	--	--

* Sample displayed pitting and the corrosion product drifted to the bottom of the test cell

Figure 4

Cyclic Polarization testing of Ti6Al4V samples as –fabricated a) Sample 1C – 90°, and b) all three orientations (both ID and OD). Pitting was verified on the samples after exposure.

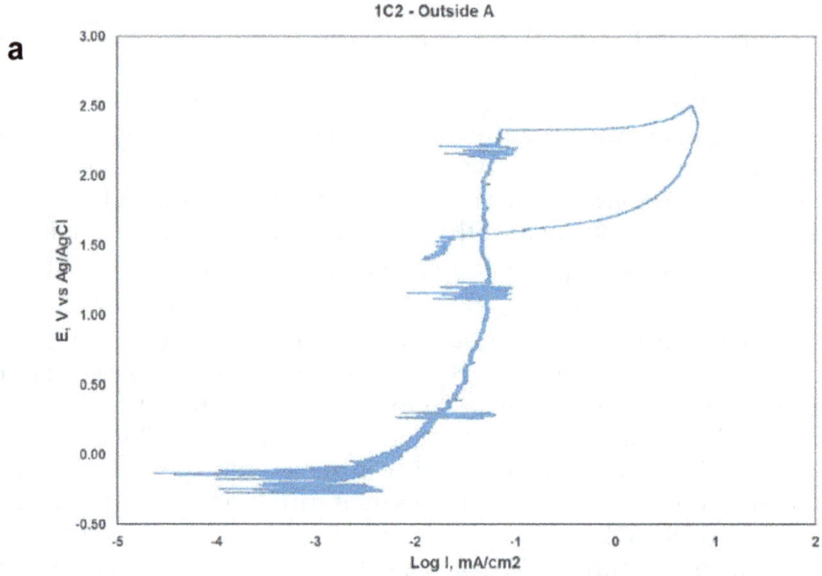

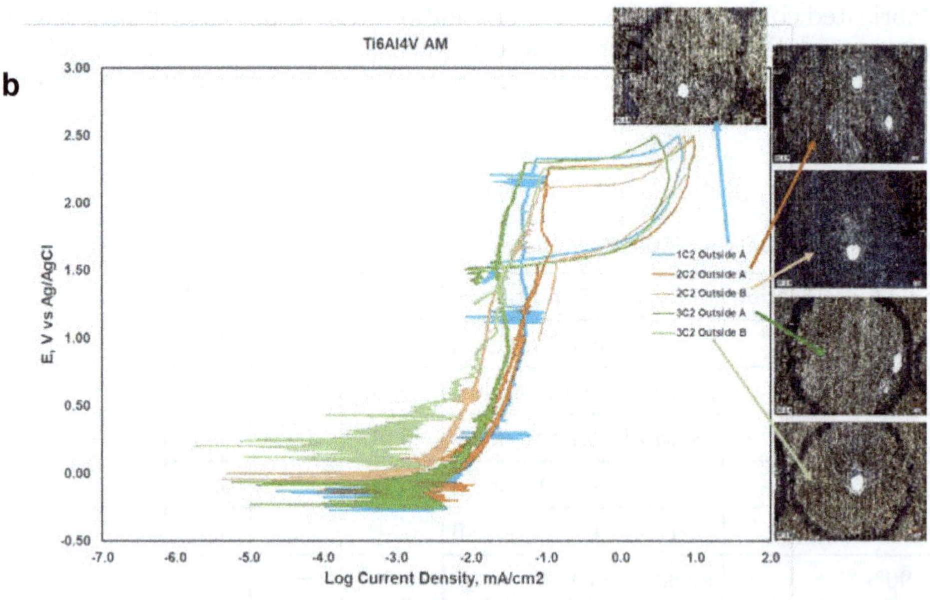

obtained in the Z direction (Figure 10a and 10b). Although the samples displayed a large current resembling transpassive behavior, the samples did not display pitting after the exposure. Thus, this increase may be due to Nickel oxidation above 1V.

Figure 5

Cyclic Polarization testing of Ti6Al4V samples as-fabricated a) polished AM samples, b) wrought Ti6Al4V and c) as-fabricated, polished and wrought conditions together. Passive currents were much lower for the polished and wrought samples, regardless of orientation.

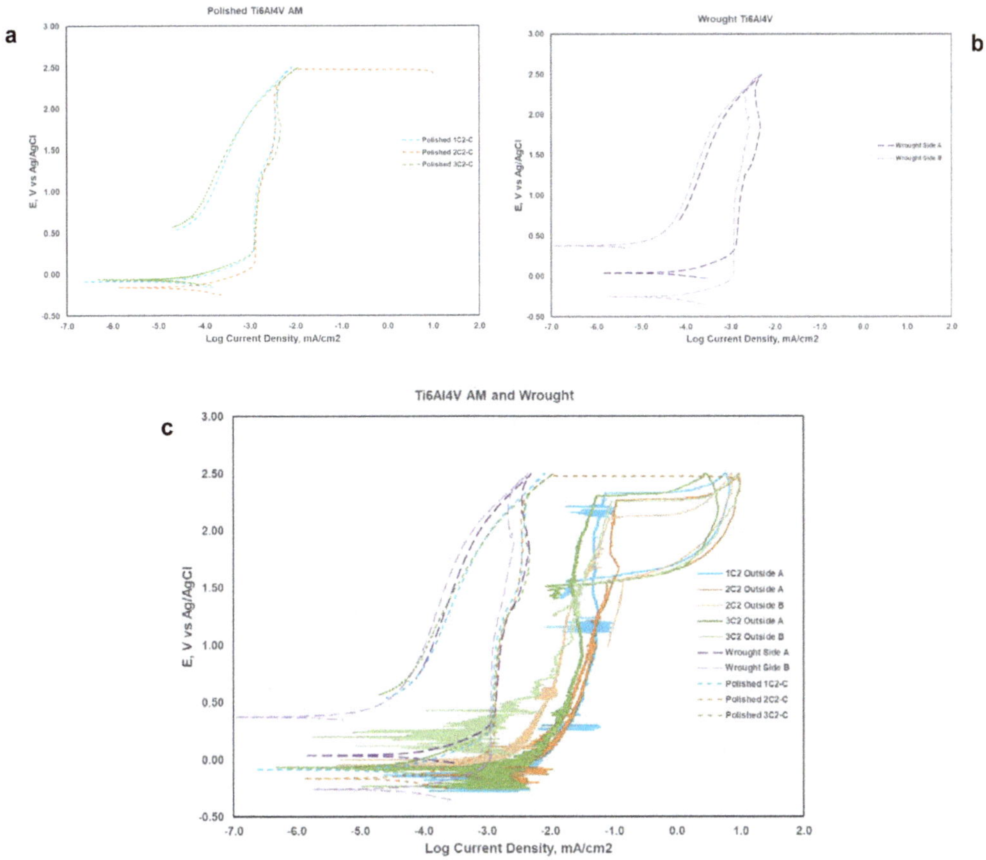

Figure 6

SEM photographs of as-fabricated Ti6Al4V 1C2 (90°) sample after CP testing a) overall pit location at 25x, and b) and c) showing crevice and corrosion locations at 1000x.

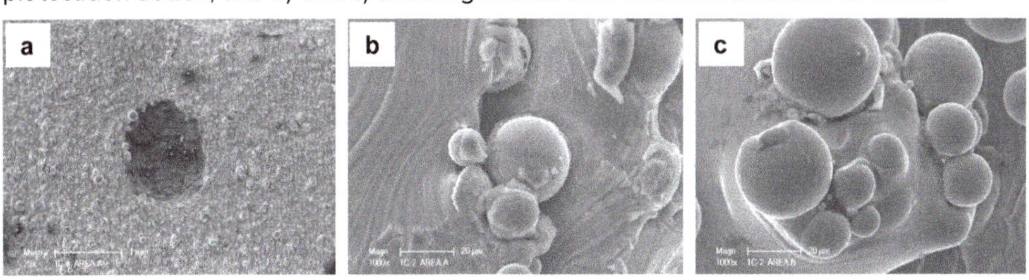

Figure 7

SEM photographs of as-fabricated Ti6Al4V 2C2 (30°) sample after CP testing a) overall pit location at 25x, and area showing crevice and corrosion locations b) at 1000x and c) at 2000x.

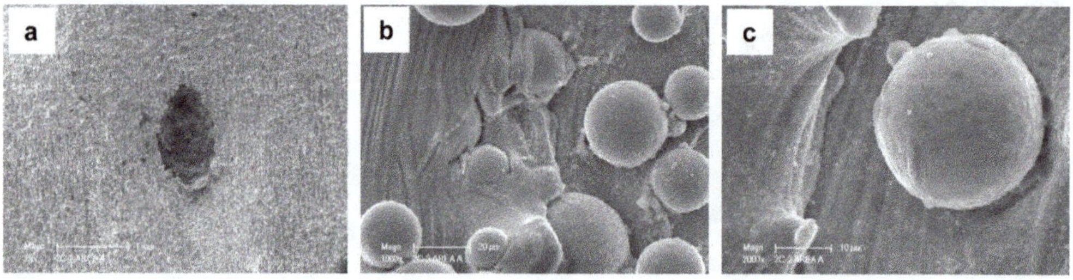

Figure 8

SEM photographs of as-fabricated Ti6Al4V 3C2 (-30°) sample after CP testing a) overall pit location at 25x, and b) and c) showing crevice and corrosion locations at 1000x.

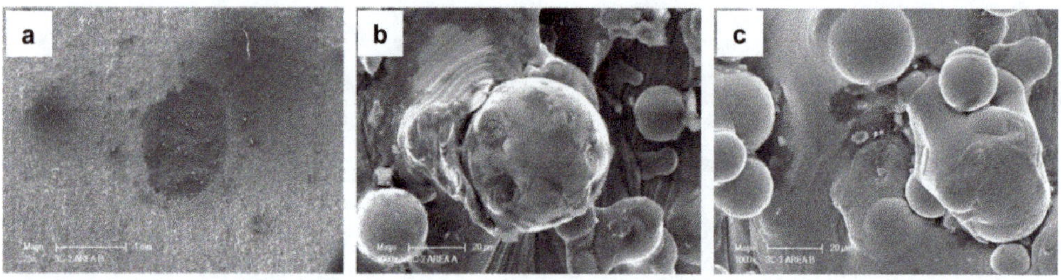

After cyclic polarization testing, there was no observable pitting on the sample surfaces, only staining of the test area. The SEM photographs also did not show preferential corrosion around the partially melted powder on the bulk surface as was seen in the Ti6Al4V. However, cracking behavior was seen on ligand type surfaces that are the result of the laser melt process as seen in Figures 11, 12, and 13.

Table 3

Surface Roughness Measurements for Nitinol Samples.

Material / Orientation	Surface Condition	Avg Ra, μm	Avg Rp, μm	Avg Rv, μm
NiTi – Z	As Fabricated	19	64	63
	Polished	0.41		
NiTi – X	As Fabricated	15	74	55
	Polished	0.49		
NiTi – Y	As Fabricated	21	58	50
	Polished	0.80		

Figure 9

SEM photographs showing surface structure of as-fabricated NiTi AM samples prior to testing in the a) Z direction, b) X direction and c) Y directions at 500x.

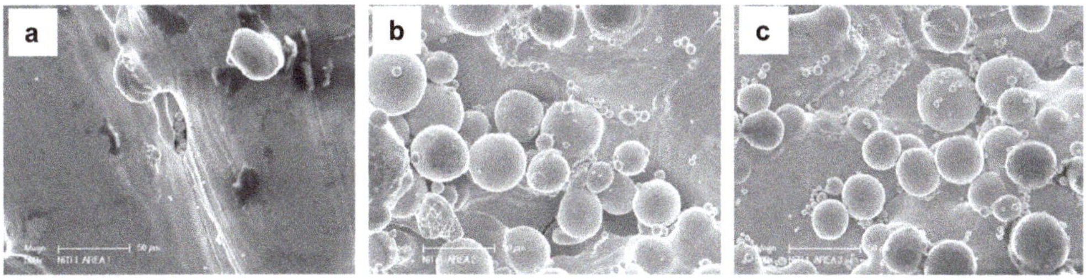

DISCUSSION

This research work reviewed the different orientations of samples during an AM build and the resulting corrosion resistance. One of the end goals of building implants using 3-D technologies is to fabricate patient specific sized implants in a minimal amount of time. Thus, it would be ideal to reduce the amount of post processing that may be required. This work has shown that the as-fabricated Ti6Al4V AM samples did not show differences in corrosion behavior in the different build orientations with regards to the coater direction (90°, 30°, and -30°). All as-fabricated samples showed higher passive currents along with disturbances in the passive region. Preferential corrosion was observed on crevices that formed due to the partial melting of the powder on the bulk surface. Polishing the sample reduced the passive currents and increased the pitting potential. Thus, the polishing step would be of great benefit for Ti6Al4V implants in terms of corrosion resistance, though it may add on additional time constructing a final product. In addition, since all three orientations showed similar behavior in the polished form were comparable to wrought Ti6Al4V, which indicated that using the entire build plate during SLM AM processing may be possible without negative corrosion consequences.

The NiTi sample also displayed some disruptions in the passive region in all three orientations (Z, X and Y). In this instance no preferential crevice corrosion, or pitting was observed after CP testing, but several areas on the tested sample surfaces showed cracking. After polishing, the samples all drifted to the lower passive current densities as was observed on the as-fabricated Z direction sample. Polishing the sample once

Table 4

Cyclic Polarization Data for NiTi Sample.

Sample Identification	Surface Condition	Eocp, V	Epit, V	Erp, V
H20-1 Z Direction	As Fabricated	0.04	--	1.01
H20-1 Z Direction	Polished	-0.135	--	0.956
H20-1 X Direction	As Fabricated	-0.022	--	1.08
H20-1 X Direction	Polished	-0.136	--	0.986
H20-1 Y Direction	As Fabricated	0.084	--	1.09
H20-1 Y Direction	Polished	-0.084	--	0.972

Figure 10

Cyclic Polarization testing of NiTi samples for the a) as-fabricated samples, b) polished samples and c) as-fabricated, and polished conditions together. Passive currents were much lower for the polished samples, regardless of orientation.

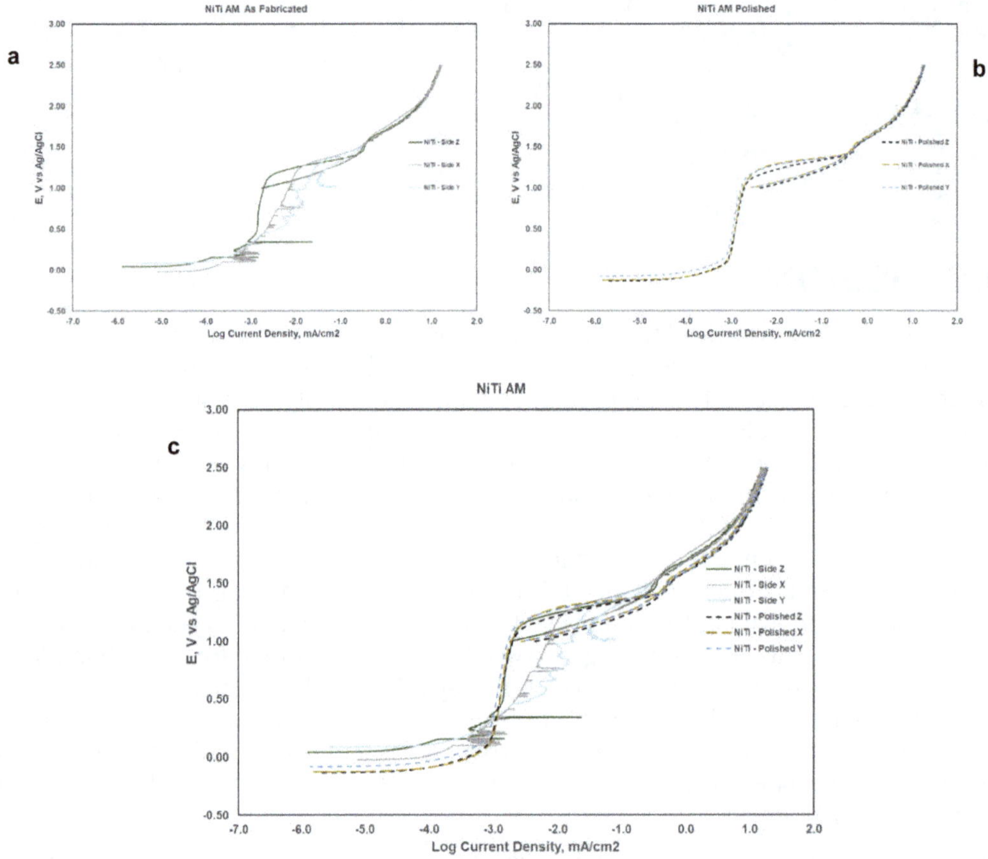

Figure 11

SEM photographs of as-fabricated NiTi Z direction sample after CP testing a) low magnification at 100x, and b) and c) showing cracking behavior of surface ligands at 1000x.

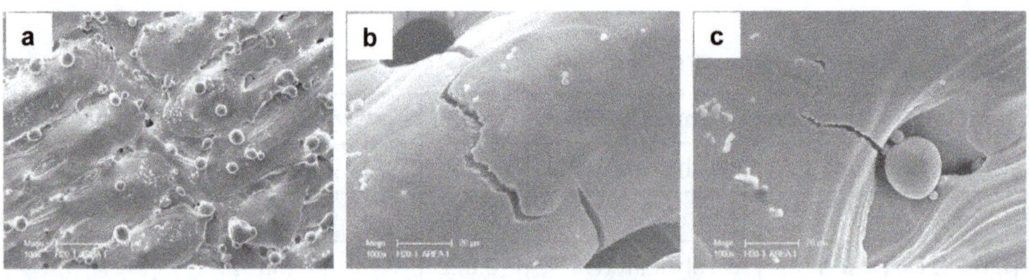

again, improved the corrosion resistance, regardless of surface orientation. There was a sharp increase in the as-fabricated and polished NiTi samples after the observed passive regions, which occurred above 1V. This may be due to Ni oxidation as there was no observed pitting on the samples after test.

Figure 12

SEM photographs of as-fabricated NiTi X direction sample after CP testing a) low magnification at 100x, and b) and c) showing cracking behavior of surface ligands at 1000x.

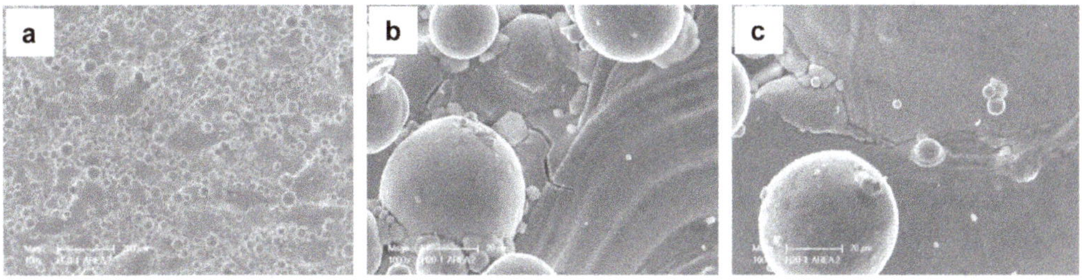

Figure 13

SEM photographs of as-fabricated NiTi Y direction sample after CP testing a) low magnification at 100x, and b) and c) showing surface ligands at with partially melted powders 1000x and 500x, respectively.

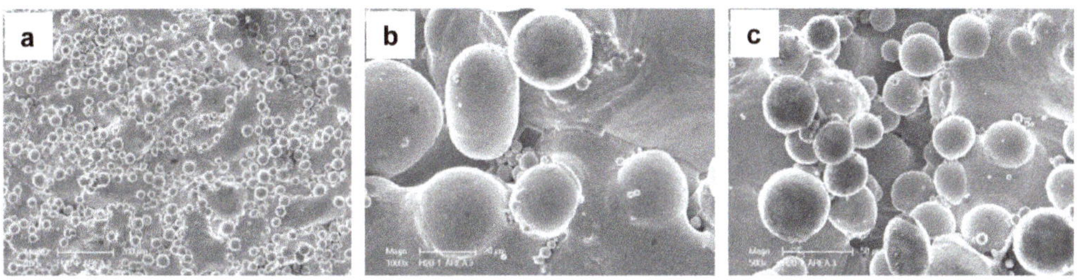

Although in both these material cases the post processing step of polishing improved corrosion resistance, other research has shown that increasing surface roughness may increase the cell adhesion on an implant surface. Utilizing the AM processing technology will then require careful consideration on what implant conditions would require, in order to consider what post processing steps would be needed, if any.

CONCLUSIONS

Cyclic polarization testing on AM fabricated Ti6Al4V and Nitinol have showed the following observations:

1. The as-fabricated Ti6Al4V cyclic polarization showed high passive currents with disturbances in the passive region. There were slight differences in the different orientations and between replicates. The pitting potentials were between 2.09 V and 2.31 V and the repassivation potential was approximately 1.5 V for all three directions. Pitting was observed on the sample after testing. SEM analysis showed preferential corrosion observed on crevices that formed due to the partial melting of the powder on the bulk surface.
2. The polished and wrought Ti6Al4V samples all showed much lower passive currents and did not show disturbances in the passive region. The pitting potential was 2.48 V for one sample and the other two samples had a E_{pit} > 2.5 V.

3. The as-fabricated Nitinol samples also showed disturbances in the passive region for all three orientations. No pitting was observed on the samples after testing, only dark staining. The SEM analysis showed that there was cracking on some of the melted AM surface ligament structures.
4. Polished AM Nitinol samples also showed much lower passive currents than the as-fabricated samples. No pitting was observed on the samples after testing.
5. For the Ti6Al4V and Nitinol samples evaluated, the three build orientations did not show appreciable differences in surface roughness or in passive current densities in the as-fabricated state. Polishing the samples, however, improved the corrosion resistance in each of the build orientations and directions. This implies that the AM build orientation does not have a measurable impact on the corrosion resistance in this instance, but additional post processing techniques such as polishing may be required to improve corrosion resistance of AM fabricated implants.

ACKNOWLEDGMENTS

The authors would like to thank the technical staff at Southwest Research Institute (Jaime Garza, Byron Chapa, Christopher Wolfe, Taylor Bartholomew, Brian Derby, and Steve Clay) for their contributions to the testing portion of this research effort.

REFERENCES

1. ASTM F2129, Standard Test Method for Conducting Cyclic Potentiodynamic Polarization Measurements to Determine the Corrosion Susceptibility of Implant Devices, 2015.
2. Murr L.E., Gaytan S.M., Ramirez D.A., Martinez E., Hernandez J., Amato K.N., Shindo P.W., Medina F.R., Wicker R.B., "Metal Fabrication by Additive Manufacturing Using Laser and Electron Beam Melting Technologies," *J. Mater. Sci. Technol.* 28, 1 (2012): p. 1.
3. Frazier W.E., "Metal Additive Manufacturing: A Review," *J. Mater. Eng. & Performance* 23, 6 (2014): p. 1917.
4. D'Urso P., Earwaker W., Barker T., Redmond M., Thompson R., Effeney D., and Tomlinson F., Custom cranioplasty using stereolithography and acrylic *Br J Plast Surg*. 53:200–204, 2000.
5. Singare S., Liu Y., Li D., Lu B., Wang J., and He S., Individually prefabricated prosthesis for maxilla reconstruction *J Prosthodont*. 17:135–140, 2008.
6. Lee M., Chang C., and Ku Y., New layer-based imaging and rapid prototyping techniques for computer-aided design and manufacture of custom dental restoration *J Med Eng Technol*. 32:83–90, 2008.
7. Dai K., Yan M., Zhu Z., and Sun Y., Computer-aided custom-made hemipelvic prosthesis used in extensive pelvic lesions *J Arthroplasty*. 22:981-986, 2007.
8. Harrysson O., Hosni Y., and Nayfeh J., Custom-designed orthopedic implants evaluated using finite element analysis of patient-specific computed tomography data: femoral-component case study *BMC Musculoskelet Disord*. 8:91, 2007.
9. He J., Li D., Lu B., Wang Z., and Tao Z., Custom fabrication of composite tibial hemi-knee joint combining CAD/CAE/CAM techniques. *Proc Inst Mech Eng*. [H] 220:823–830, 2006.

10. Wang Z., Teng Y., and Li D., Fabrication of custom-made artificial semi-knee joint based on rapid prototyping technique: computer assisted design and manufacturing *Chinese Journal of Reparative and Reconstructive Surgery* 18:347–351, 2004.
11. Murr L.E., Quinones S.A., Gaytan S.M., Lopez M.I., Rodela A., Martinez E.Y., Hernandez D.H., Martinez E., Medina F., and Wicker R.B., Microstructure and mechanical behavior of Ti–6Al–4V produced by rapid-layer manufacturing, for biomedical applications, *Journal of The Mechanical Behavior of Biomedical Materials*, 2:20-32, 2009.
12. Hamu G.B., Patient Specific Orthopedic Implants Manufactured by Additive Manufacturing – A Corrosion Study, Corrosion / 2017, Paper No. 9257.
13. Mah D., Pelletier M.H., Louric V., and Walsh W.R., *Anals of Biomed. Eng*, Vol 47, No. 1: 162-173, 2019.
14. Rahman Z., Pompa L., Haider W., Influence of Electropolishing and Magnetoelectropolishing on Corrosion and Biocompatibility of Titanium Implants, *Journal of Mat. Eng. and Performance*, 23: 3907-3915, 2014.
15. Cao L. and Paindre A., Characterization of Corrosion Behavior on Additive Manufacturing Alloys, Corrosion / 2017, Paper No. 9472.
16. Sullivan S.J.L., Madamba D., Sivan S., Miyahiro K., Dreher M.L., Trepanier C., Nagaraja S., The Effects of Surface Processing on in-vivo Corrosion of Nitinol Stents in a Porcine Model, *Acta Biomaterialia*, 2017.

Paper Number:
C2023-19413

Corrosion Behavior Assessment and Comparison of UNS S31603 Stainless Steel, Nickel-titanium Shape Memory Alloy, and $Al_2Cr_5Cu_5Fe_{53}Ni_{35}$ High-entropy Alloy in Biomedical Environments

Olivia Esmacher
Texas A&M University

Marcelo Paredes
Texas A&M University at Galveston

Deeparekha Narayanan
Texas A&M University

Homero Castaneda
Texas A&M University

Abstract

Electrochemical characterization was performed on near-equiatomic nickel-titanium shape memory alloy (SMA), $Al_2Cr_5Cu_5Fe_{53}Ni_{35}$ high entropy alloy (HEA), and UNS S31603 stainless steel to assess and compare the corrosion behavior and resistance of the material in simulated biomedical environments. A simulated bio-fluid (SBF) electrolyte was used to study the chemical and temperature-controlled parameters that the alloys experienced when they were exposed to corrosion conditions. Electrochemical testing, such as EIS and LPR tests, was performed to observe the response of the material under a range of conditions. Cyclic polarization tests were performed on all three materials to determine and compare passive to active behavior. Different performance vs. conditions correlations were described by using high-resolution surface techniques such as SEM following electrochemical testing resulting in some interfacial active-passive mechanisms.

Keywords: Alloys, EIS, Atmospheric corrosion, Polarization, Pitting corrosion

INTRODUCTION

Materials selection in the biomedical sector has become a critical area of research, and the care and treatment of patients need to be continuously improved as technology advances. There is a broad range of such applications for metals in the current state of the industry, including dentistry and orthodontics, surgical tools, implants, stents, and bone staples and screws. Each of these applications entails a unique environment within the human body, and as new alloys are developed, it is crucial to understand their degradation behavior and response when exposed to the harsh conditions found throughout biomedical applications.

For this study, three materials were selected in order to compare corrosion behavior – UNS S31603 stainless steel was chosen as a benchmark material, as it is commonly used throughout the biomedical industry for its biocompatibility and stable performance when exposed to biological environments. UNS S31603 stainless steel finds wide usage due to its good mechanical properties, versatility in shaping for different applications, and cost in comparison to other alloys. However, its chromium and nickel content necessitate a high degree of corrosion resistance to improve its longevity and control and prevent the release of potentially harmful ions into the body. Additionally, studies have shown the corrosion resistance of UNS S31603 stainless steel in biological environments is highly sensitive to surface finish, leading to more complex manufacturing methods [1, 2]. The NiTi SMA used in this study was a 55.8 wt.% Ni-rich NiTi alloy. The passive film formed on NiTi SMAs has been shown to consist of predominantly titanium oxide (TiO_2), [3] which has been shown to be stable and protect against the oxidation of Ni, making it another good choice for biocompatible implant material. The non-negligible Ni-content in these SMAs has raised some concerns about potentially harmful nickel ion release into the body, necessitating careful control of the alloy content and surface finish in order to preferentially form the biocompatible titanium oxide passive layer.

In recent years, research on high-entropy alloys (HEAs) has allowed new alloys to be developed to explore the effect of composition on mechanical behavior and interaction with the environment. These alloys are often also referred to as multi-principal element alloys (MPEAs) or complex-concentrated alloys (CCAs), and were first proposed in 2004 by Cantor et al. [4] and Yeh et al. [5, 6]. Initially, the definition of HEAs specified compounds of five or more principal elements in equimolar ratios, however, this definition has expanded over the years to include alloys with multiple principal alloying elements in a wider range of concentrations with possessing a high configurational entropy resulting in a single-phase alloy [5-9].

One of the goals of this study was to evaluate the behavior and response of a newly developed HEA material in simulated biological environments. This alloy system, $Al_2Cr_5Cu_5Fe_{53}Ni_{35}$, is expected to show passive behavior due to the passivity response of its individual elements. This novel HEA has not been widely studied in terms of electrochemical response, in relation to more conventional alloys such as UNS S31603 and Nitinol in a biological environment. In this environment, three alloys were tested and compared the differences in terms of active-passive behavior. The HEA $Al_2Cr_5Cu_5Fe_{53}Ni_{35}$ tended to form chromium and iron-rich corrosion product films, but it is not clear what particular mechanisms influence the forming of specific passive films in different environments.

EXPERIMENTAL PROCEDURE

The UNS S31603 samples were received as rod stock, which were then cut to form thin disks, cold mounted, and polished to achieve a mirror finish before being exposed to the testing solution. The NiTi SMA samples were cut from thin sheet stock into 1 cm x 1 cm squares using a slow gravity-fed cutter in order to reduce temperature fluctuations in the material during processing. The samples were then cold mounted in epoxy and polished to mirror finish before testing.

The $Al_2Cr_5Cu_5Fe_{53}Ni_{35}$ high entropy alloy is a newly developed alloy that has not been previously tested for biological environments. In studies of this material in other chloride-containing solutions, it has been shown to produce Al_2O_3 and Cr_2O_3 as its most common corrosion products [10]. The samples were received in rod stock and cut to form thin disks with 1 cm diameter, cold mounted and polished to mirror finish. The composition of all testing samples can be found in Table 1.

The testing solution chosen for this study was Simulated Body-Fluid (SBF), which is commonly used in biomedical experiments to simulate conditions of the human body, specifically environments containing blood plasma. The solution was prepared according to protocol found in literature [11] and the excess solution stored in refrigerated conditions until additional required for additional experiments. The solution ion concentration can be seen in Table 2.

All experiments were performed in a jacketed electrochemical testing cell, allowing coolant to flow around the solution at a set temperature of 37°C, and the solution was exposed to ambient air. The samples were tested by using different techniques. All tests were carried out using a standard three-electrode cell and a potentiostat, with a graphite counter electrode and Ag/AgCl reference electrode. Before all tests, the open circuit potential (OCP) was monitored for 60 minutes in order to allow the sample to stabilize in its environment.

Cyclic polarization tests were performed to determine the material's passivity response and pitting behavior, generating cathodic and anodic polarization curves with a forward scan of -150 mV related to OCP at a scan rate of 1 mV/s to an apex of 1.5 V relative to OCP before reversing the scan direction until reaching OCP. Electrochemical impedance spectroscopy (EIS) was performed in both short term (single run) tests and long-term immersion tests (completed hourly for a period of 7 days) to observe the initial and dynamic passive behavior of these materials over longer exposure to simulated biological conditions.

In order to observe changes in the material conditions after testing was performed, microstructural characterization was performed including scanning electron microscopy (SEM) and energy-dispersive spectroscopy (EDS) in order to identify the corrosion products.

Table 1

Nominal composition of as-received samples (wt%) [1, 3, 10].

	Cr	Ni	Mn	Si	P	S	Mo	Fe	Cu	Ti	Al
UNS S31603	18%	10%	2%	1%	0.05%	0.03%	2.5%	66.42%	N/A	N/A	N/A
HEA	5%	35%	N/A	N/A	N/A	N/A	N/A	53%	5%	N/A	2%
SMA	<0.01%	55.8%	N/A	N/A	N/A	N/A	N/A	<0.05%	<0.01%	44.2%	N/A

Table 2

Ion concentration (mM) for Simulated Body Fluid (SBF).

Ion	Simulated Body Fluid (SBF)
Na^+	142.0
K^+	5.0
Mg^{2+}	1.5
Ca^{2+}	2.5
Cl^-	148.8
HCO_3^-	4.2
HPO_4^{2-}	1.0
SO_4^{2-}	0.5

Figure 1

Cyclic polarization plot for NiTi SMA (blue), UNS S31603 (orange), and HEA (green) in SBF.

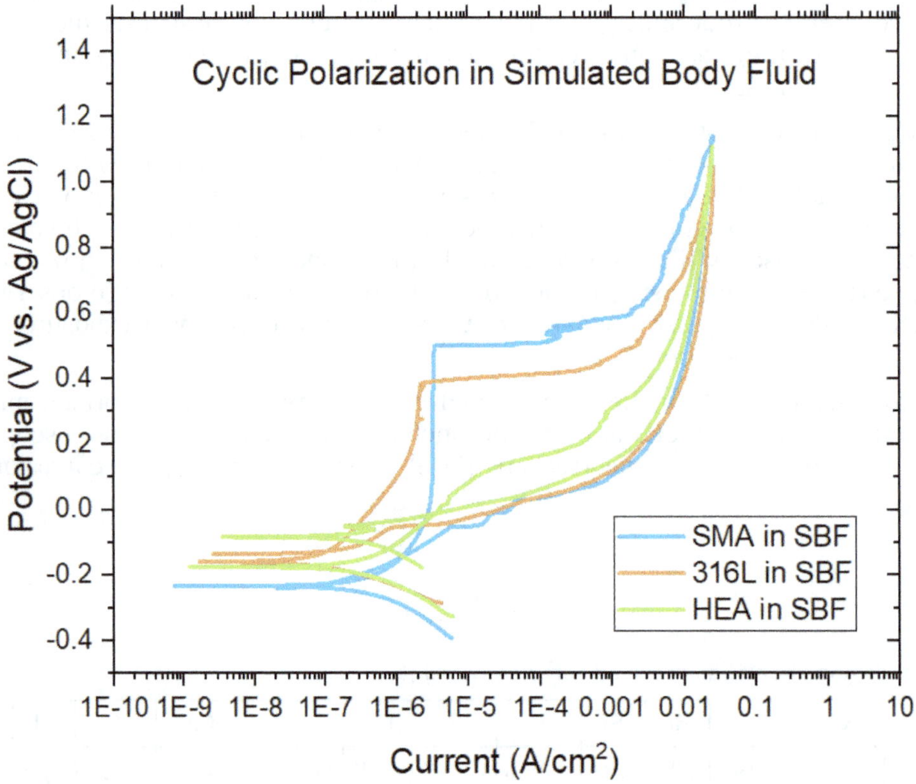

RESULTS

Cyclic Polarization Tests – SBF

Figure 1 below shows the cyclic polarization plots for the SMA (blue), UNS S31603 (orange), and HEA (green) material samples in SBF. The corrosion parameters obtained from these tests are found in Table 3.

Cyclic polarization testing of the three materials in SBF at body temperature revealed that in comparison to the UNS S31603 benchmark sample, the SMA sample showed similar passive behavior, while the HEA sample did not show strong evidence of

Table 3

Corrosion parameters calculated from cyclic polarization testing for NiTi SMA, UNS S31603, and HEA in SBF.

Sample	E_b (V)	E_{rev} (V)	E_{rep} (V)	Passive Region (V)	Pitting Region (V)
NiTi	0.5	1.15	-0.12	0.5	0.65
UNS S31603	0.4	1.05	-0.11	0.2	0.65
HEA	0.1	1.1	0	N/A	1

Figure 2

Phase angle (left), and Nyquist (right) plots for NiTi SMA as observed during EIS testing during immersion in SBF for 1 week.

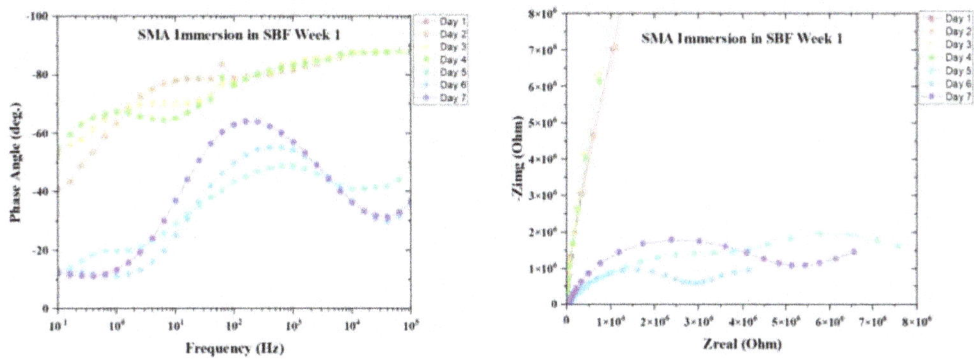

passivity under these conditions. The passive region for the SMA sample showed a slightly larger passive region (area where change in corrosion current is minimal) and very similar pitting region (area between passive layer breakdown and reverse scan voltage) than the UNS S31603. The voltage of passive layer breakdown (denoted E_b) was very similar for the SMA and UNS S31603. All of the materials displayed positive hysteresis and evidence of pitting potential.

Immersion Tests - SMA In SBF for 7 Days

Figure 2 shows the evolution of the response of the SMA sample over 7 days continuous exposure in SBF. In the early testing period, the phase angle and Nyquist radius show an increase with time, indicating a passive layer formed on the sample surface. This trend is less clearly pronounced in the phase angle after the 2nd day of immersion, indicating a metastable oxide layer that is beginning to become more porous and allowing dissolution of the layer into the solution. In the latter half of the testing period, the behavior changes, showing a marked decrease in the semicircle shape of the Nyquist plot, as well as a single time constant peak in the phase angle and significantly lower magnitude at low frequency (about 10 Hz) of around 10-15 degrees. This is indicative of an increase in porosity of the passive film, allowing solution uptake to occur, changing the capacitance behavior of the material over time.

Immersion Tests - HEA in SBF for 7 Days

Figure 3 shows the HEA signature, at early times the phase angle shows at lower frequency (around 10 Hz) a magnitude of 75 degrees and decreases afterwards. At mid frequencies the phase angle shows the formation of one time constant at mid-frequency and fluctuating at around 50 Hz and just below 60 degrees. The low frequency denotes the interface between the metallic sample and how the charge transfer is decreasing, this latter due to the corrosion products porosity and the capacitive like behavior at the interface. The Nyquist diagram shows fluctuating behavior, with a general decrease in the semicircle shape with time, this latter reinforces the interfacial mechanism governing the system. The corrosion products forming at the interface following the dissolution process influence the capacitance like behavior and also the charge transfer resistance magnitude due to the dissolution of the surface in this electrolyte.

Immersion Tests - UNS S31603 in SBF for 7 Days

Figure 3

Phase angle (left), and Nyquist (right) plots for HEA as observed during EIS testing during immersion in SBF for 1 week.

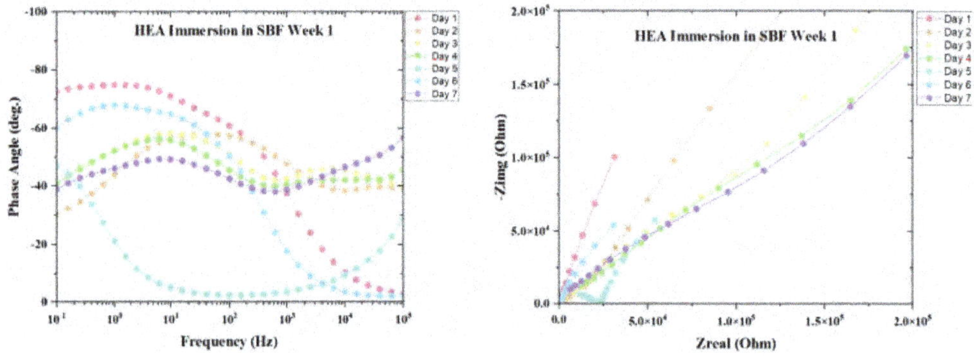

Figure 4

Phase angle (left), and Nyquist (right) plots for UNS S31603 as observed during EIS testing during immersion in SBF for 1 week.

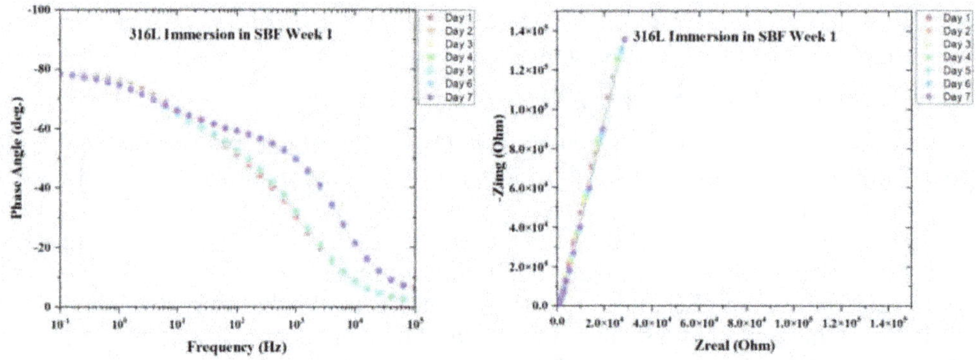

Figure 4 shows the response of the UNS S31603 sample throughout 7 days of immersion in SBF. The UNS S31603 sample showed significantly higher stability across the testing duration compared to the other two materials, with small variation in the corrosion resistance with time. The time constant observed at low frequency (around 10 Hz) has a magnitude of 80 degrees and shows evidence of a compact, stable passive film formed on the sample surface that has little porosity and thus does not uptake solution. This behavior is consistent from the first day, with small changes in the phase angle and Nyquist response during the first 24 hours and negligible changes thereafter.

Discussion of Results

Electrochemical Testing

Figure 5 shows the corrosion resistance from fitting equivalent circuit models to the data acquired from EIS testing over 10 days immersion in SBF. As was stated in the EIS results section, the UNS S31603 (green) shows extremely consistent performance throughout the entire 10 day period, with very small fluctuations and no clear increasing or decreasing trend. While the corrosion resistance observed is of a lower

Figure 5

Corrosion resistance (R_p) of NiTi SMA (red), HEA (blue), and UNS S31603 (green) as calculated from EIS equivalent circuit fitting for testing immersed in SBF for 10 days.

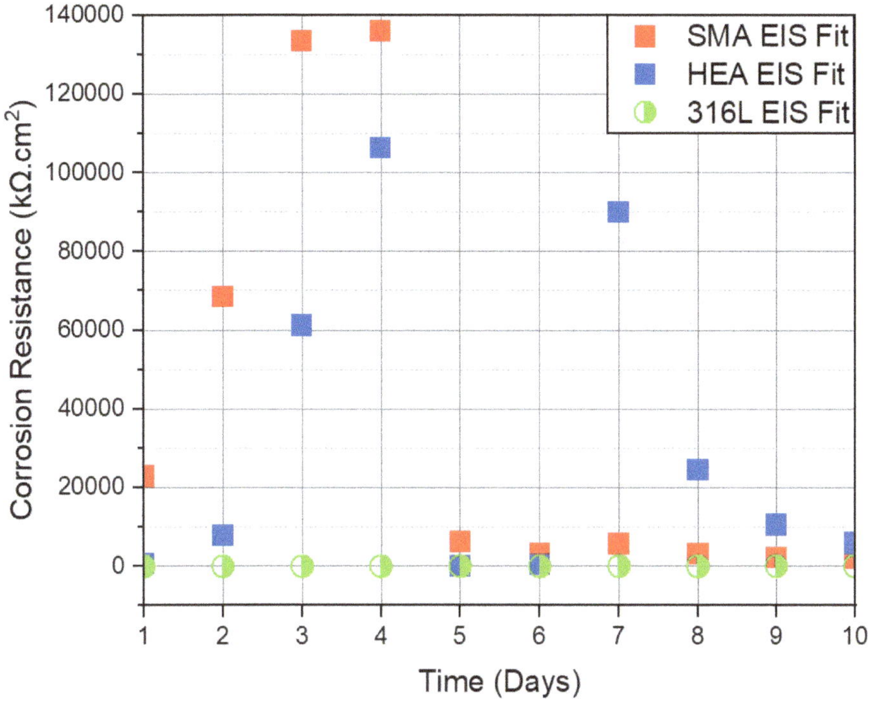

magnitude than the other two tested materials, it shows strong evidence of a very stable passive film formed on the surface of the sample, which is highly desired for reliable biocompatibility applications. In contrast, the SMA sample (red) shows a very high and increasing magnitude for the first 4 days of exposure, which then decreases sharply and stabilizes to be very similar to the UNS S31603 sample for the remainder of the testing period. This is indicative of a strong passive film growing for the initial period of the test, which is then damaged in some degree to reduce the corrosion resistance to a comparable level of the UNS S31603 benchmark material.

The HEA sample (blue) shows evidence of repassivation during the testing period, and a different corrosion behavior than the other two samples. Over the first 4 days, the corrosion resistance increases, and then decreases sharply, similarly to the trend observed in the SMA sample. However, for the HEA material, the corrosion resistance increases again after 7 days immersion, then gradually decreases the remainder of the testing period back to the same level of the other two materials. The is indicative of a strong barrier to corrosion forming during the initial testing period, a breakdown of the passive film to some degree, and then reforming and subsequent degradation of the barrier again for the remainder of the testing period. This is reflective of the behavior observed in the electrochemical testing, as well as the corrosion product observed in the surface characterization discussed in the next section.

Figure 6

SEM-EDS imaging of HEA sample surface after continuous EIS testing immersed in SBF for 2 weeks.

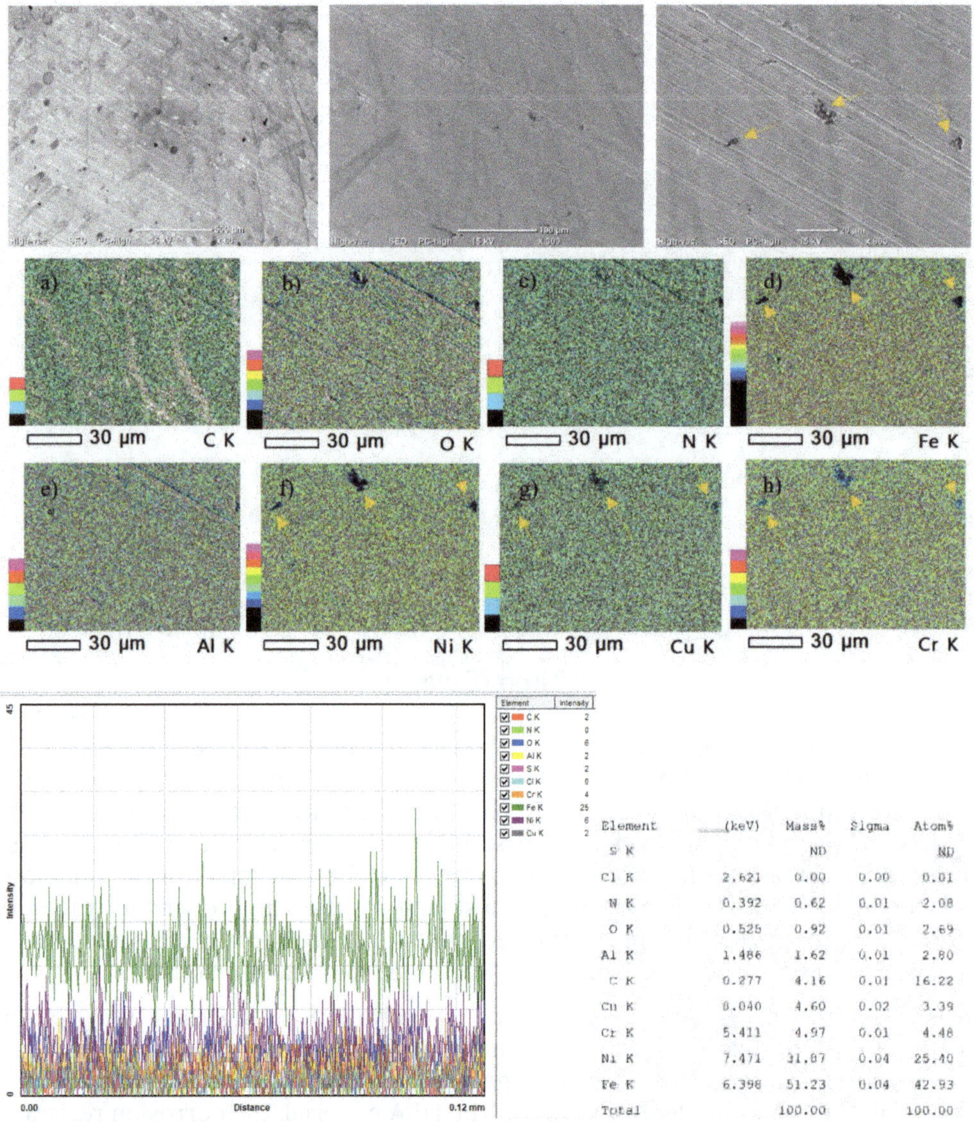

Element	(keV)	Mass%	Sigma	Atom%
S K		ND		ND
Cl K	2.621	0.00	0.00	0.01
N K	0.392	0.62	0.01	2.08
O K	0.525	0.92	0.01	2.69
Al K	1.486	1.62	0.01	2.80
C K	0.277	4.16	0.01	16.22
Cu K	8.040	4.60	0.02	3.39
Cr K	5.411	4.97	0.01	4.48
Ni K	7.471	31.87	0.04	25.40
Fe K	6.398	51.23	0.04	42.93
Total		100.00		100.00

Surface Characterization – 14 Day Immersion Testing

After sonicating in ethanol to remove surface deposits of chlorides, the HEA sample showed evidence of a film remaining on the surface in both optical microscopy and SEM imaging. Additionally, there were small portions of the sample that showed as iron oxidation product. The non-uniformity of the features implies some degree of localized attack as well as the possibility of selective leaching. In order to investigate these features further, EDS was utilized to characterize their composition.

An EDS inspection of the film feature shows deposits containing carbon from immersion in the SBF solution for two weeks, as seen in Figure 6a. EDS analysis performed on the substrate contains iron and nickel as the most abundant elements, followed by chromium, copper and aluminum. A feature observed in the SEM imaging for the HEA sample is the formation of irregularly shaped pit-like features measuring approximately 5 µm to 10 µm, which can be seen in Figure 6c. EDS analysis of these areas show a significant decrease of Fe and Ni content as indicated by the black areas in Figure 6d and 6f. These same areas show evidence of lower Cu and Cr content as well, and perhaps most notably, the Al content of the alloy appears to remain intact in these areas after immersion in SBF for two weeks. From the EDS imaging, the corrosion product around the perimeter of these irregularly shaped pit areas appears to be chromium oxide and cupric oxide, with the interior of the crater showing as aluminum from the original alloy composition.

This investigation result is particularly of importance to the observation of the corrosion behavior of this HEA, as it implies that some selective local attack is occurring in this environment. Due to the complex nature of this alloy composition, there is potential for formation of a micro-galvanic cell within the metal substrate, allowing for leaching of some elements into the solution. Additionally, coupled with the response observed in the electrochemical testing, the passive film formed on the HEA is not stable over time, and experiences breakdown and repassivation that could allow for undesired ion release of the base material or corrosion products into the body.

After removal from the SBF environment after a two-week period, the SMA sample was sonicated in ethanol to remove most of the deposits from the solution that had adhered to its surface. Upon inspection in SEM imaging, there are still very small traces of carbon deposit from the SBF on the sample surface, appearing as dark dots. At higher magnification, very small (<1µm) pits can be observed within the deposit film, identified by EDS scanning as Ti-rich areas where Ni has been removed (Figure 7e and 7f). The bulk of the surface is composed primarily of nickel and titanium, with small amounts of oxygen, carbon, chloride and sulfur deposited on the surface.

Upon removal from the SBF solution after 2 weeks, the UNS S31603 sample showed large deposits of contaminants from the solution, which were cleaned off through sonication in ethanol prior to imaging via SEM-EDS. As observed in Figure 8, the sample still retained some amount of film deposit from the solution containing carbon. Additionally, through high magnification EDS analysis of the surface area, it can be seen that there are very small (>1µm) pits appearing as black dots in which the Fe has dissolved, as well as evidence of reduced Ni and Cr content in these locations (Figure 8d, 8f and 8h). This result is similar to that observed in the SMA sample, and is indicative of the same stable passive film protecting the majority of the metallic substrate from solution uptake as seen in the electrochemical testing results.

Figure 7

SEM-EDS imaging of NiTi SMA sample surface after continuous EIS testing immersed in SBF for 2 weeks.

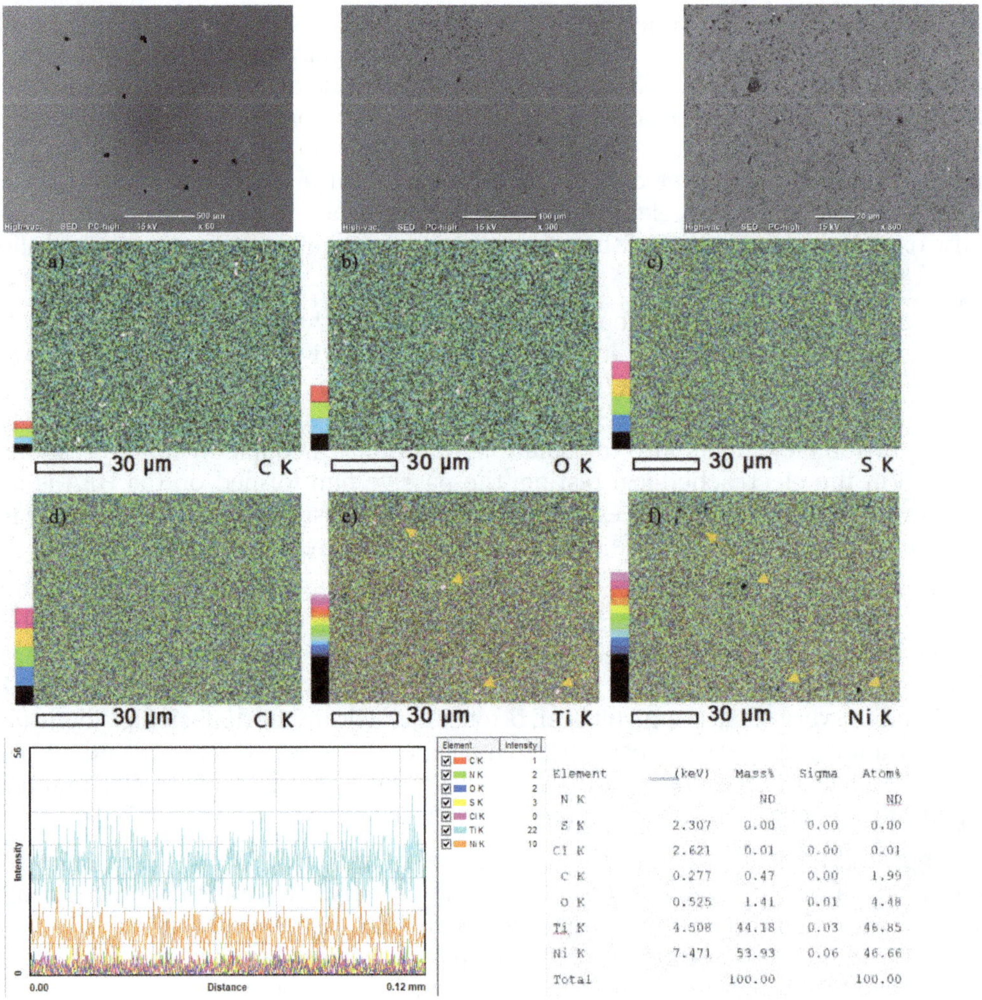

Element	(keV)	Mass%	Sigma	Atom%
N K		ND		ND
S K	2.307	0.00	0.00	0.00
Cl K	2.621	0.01	0.00	0.01
C K	0.277	0.47	0.00	1.99
O K	0.525	1.41	0.01	4.48
Ti K	4.508	44.18	0.03	46.85
Ni K	7.471	53.93	0.06	46.66
Total		100.00		100.00

Figure 8

SEM-EDS imaging of UNS S31603 sample surface after continuous EIS testing immersed in SBF for 2 weeks.

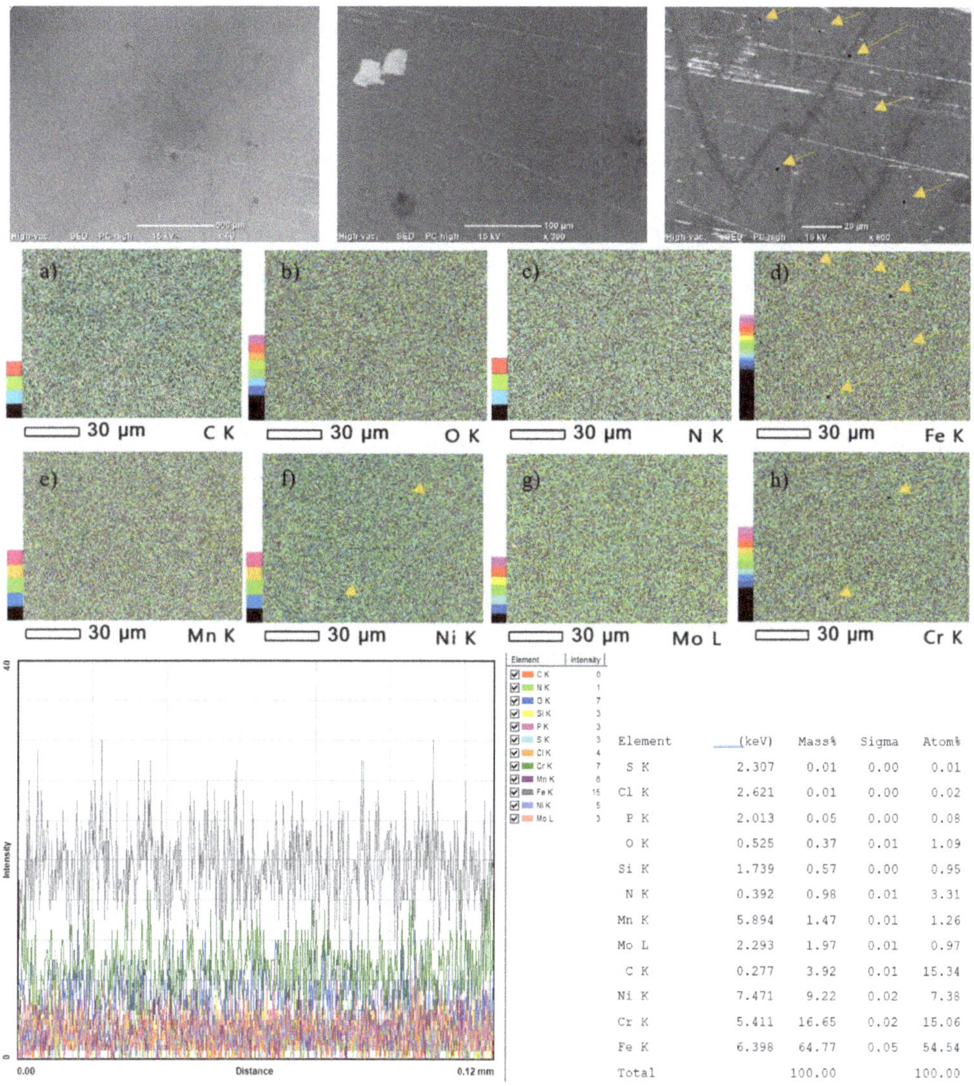

Element	(keV)	Mass%	Sigma	Atom%
S K	2.307	0.01	0.00	0.01
Cl K	2.621	0.01	0.00	0.02
P K	2.013	0.05	0.00	0.08
O K	0.525	0.37	0.01	1.09
Si K	1.739	0.57	0.00	0.95
N K	0.392	0.98	0.01	3.31
Mn K	5.894	1.47	0.01	1.26
Mo L	2.293	1.97	0.01	0.97
C K	0.277	3.92	0.01	15.34
Ni K	7.471	9.22	0.02	7.38
Cr K	5.411	16.65	0.02	15.06
Fe K	6.398	64.77	0.05	54.54
Total		100.00		100.00

CONCLUSIONS

The results of this study indicate that:

- Of the three tested materials, the HEA sample showed to be the most active under cyclic polarization testing, showing no appreciable passive region.
- The SMA and UNS S31603 samples showed very similar passivation behavior during cyclic polarization testing, with SMA having a slightly larger passive region and comparable pitting region.

- In 7-day testing, the UNS S31603 showed the most stable passive film behavior, with negligible value fluctuations. The SMA sample indicated that a very compact passive film formed during the initial test period, then broke down resulting in lower corrosion resistance with time. The HEA sample formed a compact passive film, which broke down, reformed, and broke down again. For passive film stability, UNS S31603 > SMA > HEA.
- SEM-EDS revealed after 14 days of continuous immersion the HEA sample showed evidence of localized corrosion and possible microgalvanic cell formation, while the SMA sample contained very small (>1μm) pit areas that were Ti-rich.

ACKNOWLEDGEMENTS

The authors would like to thank Dr. Marcelo Paredes and Dr. Lufeng Xue for their assistance in characterizing the HEA.

REFERENCES

1. Shih C.-C., et al., Effect of surface oxide properties on corrosion resistance of UNS S31603 stainless steel for biomedical applications. *Corrosion Science*, 2004. 46(2): p. 427-441.
2. Bordjih K., et al., Evaluation of the effect of three surface treatments on the biocompatibility of UNS S31603 stainless steel using human differentiated cells. *Biomaterials*, 1996. 17(5): p. 491-500.
3. Cisse O., et al., Effect of surface treatment of NiTi alloy on its corrosion behavior in Hanks' solution. *Journal of Biomedical Materials Research: An Official Journal of The Society for Biomaterials, The Japanese Society for Biomaterials, and The Australian Society for Biomaterials and the Korean Society for Biomaterials*, 2002. 61(3): p. 339-345.
4. Cantor B., et al., Microstructural development in equiatomic multicomponent alloys. *Materials Science and Engineering*: A, 2004. 375: p. 213-218.
5. Yeh J.W., et al., Nanostructured high-entropy alloys with multiple principal elements: novel alloy design concepts and outcomes. *Advanced engineering materials*, 2004. 6(5): p. 299-303.
6. Yeh J.-W., et al., Formation of simple crystal structures in Cu-Co-Ni-Cr-Al-Fe-Ti-V alloys with multi-principal metallic elements. *Metallurgical and Materials Transactions* A, 2004. 35(8): p. 2533-2536.
7. Chen T.-K., et al., Nanostructured nitride films of multi-element high-entropy alloys by reactive DC sputtering. *Surface and Coatings Technology*, 2005. 200(5-6): p. 1361-1365.
8. Hsu, C.-Y., et al., Wear resistance and high-temperature compression strength of Fcc CuCoNiCrAl0. 5Fe alloy with boron addition. *Metallurgical and Materials Transactions* A, 2004. 35(5): p. 1465-1469.
9. Huang P.K., et al., Multi-principal-element alloys with improved oxidation and wear resistance for thermal spray coating. *Advanced Engineering Materials*, 2004. 6(1-2): p. 74-78.
10. Xue L., et al., *Temperature and Chloride Concentration Effects on the Corrosion Behavior of Al2cr5cu5fe53ni35 High-Entropy Alloy in Marine Environment*. Available at SSRN 4032452.
11. Kokubo T., et al., Solutions able to reproduce in vivo surface-structure changes in bioactive glass-ceramic A-W. *J Biomed Mater Res*, 1990. 24(6): p. 721-734.

www.ingramcontent.com/pod-product-compliance
Lightning Source LLC
LaVergne TN
LVHW060042210926
848481LV00013B/3928